GENETICS - RESEARCH AND ISSUES

TYPE I COLLAGEN

MOLECULAR STRUCTURE, APPLICATIONS IN TISSUE ENGINEERING AND ROLE IN HUMAN DISORDERS

Genetics - Research and Issues

Additional books in this series can be found on Nova's website under the Series tab.

Additional e-books in this series can be found on Nova's website under the e-book tab.

GENETICS - RESEARCH AND ISSUES

TYPE I COLLAGEN

MOLECULAR STRUCTURE, APPLICATIONS IN TISSUE ENGINEERING AND ROLE IN HUMAN DISORDERS

GRETCHEN RIVERA
EDITOR

NOVA BIOMEDICAL
New York

Library of Congress Cataloging-in-Publication Data

ISBN: 978-1-63482-829-1

Published by Nova Science Publishers, Inc. † New York

Contents

Preface **vii**

Chapter 1 Bovine Type I Collagen: Preparation, Characterization, and Application in Tissue Regeneration **1**
Hai Lin and Yujiang Fan

Chapter 2 Structural Analyses of Type I Collagen Fibrils for Application to Tissue Engineering **73**
Koichi Morimoto and Saori Kunii

Chapter 3 Type-I Collagen Characterization of Humans Suffering Osteogenesis Imperfecta: A Skin Study by Second-Harmonic-Generation Microscopy and Texture Analysis **87**
Javier Adur, Lilia D'Souza-Li, Hernandes F. Carvalho, Carlos L. Cesar and Víctor H. Casco

Index **117**

Preface

In this book, the preparation, characterization and applications in tissue regeneration of bovine type 1 collagen are reviewed. Furthermore, collagen is often used in regenerative medicine. In this book, the authors report on the helicity of collagen molecule in fibrils by circular dichroism spectroscopy and the thermograph of fibrils by differential scanning calorimetry (the structural aspects of collagen molecules). In the last chapter, second harmonic generation (SHG) microscopy is reviewed and its potential to visualize collagen fibers in a variety of connective tissues.

Chapter 1 – In the human body, collagen is the most abundant structural protein, forming up to 35% of the entire protein content of the whole body. Type I collagen, as the main collagen in various connective tissues, presents mostly in fibrous tissues such as skin, ligaments, and tendons. Type I collagen is also related to wound healing, and is frequently found in scar tissues as well as tissues formed through reparative processes. Heterogeneous type I collagen, which possesses similar structural characters with human type I collagen, shows outstanding biocompatibility and potential bioactivity. As a natural product, it is considered to have favorable biological properties that artificial materials do not have. Therefore, it was employed as ideal biomaterials in many medical applications. In recent decades, the research on the application of type I collagen in tissue regeneration was blooming and lots of achievements were reported.

In this chapter, the preparation, characterization, and application in tissue regeneration of bovine type I collagen were reviewed with recent literatures and the authors' own studies. The preparation process of bovine type I collagen was divided into three stages: pretreatment stage, extraction stage, and purification stage. The features of these three stages were introduced and the processes were described accordingly. The problems most frequently encountered during the preparation process were illustrated, mainly based on the authors' research. According to the standards issued by ASTM and ISO, the characterization of bovine type I collagen was introduced. Meanwhile, the arguments on the risk of animal-derived starting materials for tissue engineering medical products were presented.

The application of bovine type I collagen in tissue regeneration ranging from 2D materials, such as surface coatings and thin membranes, to 3D tissue scaffolds such as sponges and hydrogels, were then summarized, focusing on the recent progress in the latest decade. The classification of biomaterials derived from bovine type I collagen was briefly reviewed according to fabrication approaches. Their state of the art clinic application in reparation and regeneration of bone, skin, ligament, etc. were introduced with focusing on the collagen-based hydrogels in cartilage defect reconstruction. Furthermore, the recent improvements on collagen fundamental researches, based on the studies trying to uncover the intriguing roles of collagen in cell-material interactions, were also introduced.

Chapter 2 – Type I collagen molecules spontaneously form insoluble fibrils at physiological buffers and at neutral pH. Insoluble fibrils play an important role in not only structure stabilization in tissue but also maintenance of each cell. Recently, collagen has been used as one of cell scaffolds in regenerative medicine. In cell culture conditions, the structure of molecule in collagen fibrils would be different from that of collagen monomer. Then, the study in ultrastructure of fibril is more important than that of monomer to understand cell behaviors. However, the structural information is not well understood yet. In this Chapter, the authors report on the helicity of collagen molecule in fibrils by circular dichroism spectroscopy and the thermograph of fibrils by differential scanning calorimetry. Furthermore, they observed the appearance of mouse neutrophil on collagen scaffolds showing imperfect fibrils. The authors' data indicated that the ultrastructure of collagen molecule depends on monomer or fibrils. The authors suggest that the formation of collagen fibrils prior to cell seeding is necessary for the interaction between cells and extracellular matrices.

Chapter 3 – *Osteogenesis imperfecta* (OI) composes a group of inherited connective tissue disorders, mainly characterized by bone fragility. It is primarily caused by mutations in the genes coding for pro-α1 and pro-α2 chains of type I collagen. The primary OI clinical manifestation is related to defective bone type I collagen fibers, although the condition is also displayed in other type I collagen-containing tissues, as skin. This means that the disease signature (collagen fibrils abnormally organized, oddly small, or both) could be readily detected in skin, which is more accessible than bone for ex vivo analysis. The molecular diagnosis of OI is nowadays based on laborious and time-consuming biochemical and/or histological methods, to evaluate the collagen from biopsy-derived dermal fibroblasts. Therefore, there is a clear need to develop a rapid noninvasive method to diagnose OI.

Second Harmonic Generation (SHG) has emerged as a powerful nonlinear optical contrast mechanism with potential to visualize collagen fibers in a variety of connective tissues. SHG signals depend on non-linear interactions of light with a sub-micron noncentrosymmetric environment. Due to the type of fibrillar structure, collagen is one of the major sources of such signals in biological materials. The aim of the present chapter is to show that SHG microscopy, in combination with appropriated quantification methods, applied to human skin provides an OI diagnostic tool to discriminate diseased from normal tissues. Moreover, this method provides a fine tone approach to differentiate clinical sub-types of OI disorders, being highly advantageous over present primarily clinical diagnostic methods, providing fast and clear confirmation.

In: Type I Collagen
Editor: Gretchen Rivera

ISBN: 978-1-63482-829-1

Chapter 1

Bovine Type I Collagen: Preparation, Characterization, and Application in Tissue Regeneration

Hai Lin and Yujiang Fan *
National Engineering Research Center for Biomaterials,
Sichuan University, Chengdu, China

Abstract

In the human body, collagen is the most abundant structural protein, forming up to 35% of the entire protein content of the whole body. Type I collagen, as the main collagen in various connective tissues, presents mostly in fibrous tissues such as skin, ligaments, and tendons. Type I collagen is also related to wound healing, and is frequently found in scar tissues as well as tissues formed through reparative processes. Heterogeneous type I collagen, which possesses similar structural characters with human type I collagen, shows outstanding bio-compatibility and potential bioactivity. As a natural product, it is considered to have favorable biological properties that artificial materials do not have. Therefore, it was employed as ideal biomaterials in many

* Corresponding author: Yujiang Fan, Tel: +86-28-85416196; Fax: +86-28-85410246. E-mail: fan_yujiang@scu.edu.cn.

medical applications. In recent decades, the research on the application of type I collagen in tissue regeneration was blooming and lots of achievements were reported.

In this chapter, the preparation, characterization, and application in tissue regeneration of bovine type I collagen were reviewed with recent literatures and our own studies. The preparation process of bovine type I collagen was divided into three stages: pretreatment stage, extraction stage, and purification stage. The features of these three stages were introduced and the processes were described accordingly. The problems most frequently encountered during the preparation process were illustrated, mainly based on our research. According to the standards issued by ASTM and ISO, the characterization of bovine type I collagen was introduced. Meanwhile, the arguments on the risk of animal-derived starting materials for tissue engineering medical products were presented.

The application of bovine type I collagen in tissue regeneration ranging from 2D materials, such as surface coatings and thin membranes, to 3D tissue scaffolds such as sponges and hydrogels, were then summarized, focusing on the recent progress in the latest decade. The classification of biomaterials derived from bovine type I collagen was briefly reviewed according to fabrication approaches. Their state of the art clinic application in reparation and regeneration of bone, skin, ligament, etc. were introduced with focusing on the collagen-based hydrogels in cartilage defect reconstruction. Furthermore, the recent improvements on collagen fundamental researches, based on the studies trying to uncover the intriguing roles of collagen in cell-material interactions, were also introduced.

Keywords: collagen type I; preparation; characterization; biosafety; scaffold; tissue engineering

1. Introduction

Collagen is an abundant structural protein of the various connective tissues in all animals. In human, the collagen accounts for about 35% of the entire protein content of the whole body. Up to twenty-nine different types of collagen have been identified and described [1]. Among the various collagen types, the type I collagen is paid great attention since it is highly contained in connective tissues and easily available under controllable techniques, leading to its wide use in the research environments and medical applications.

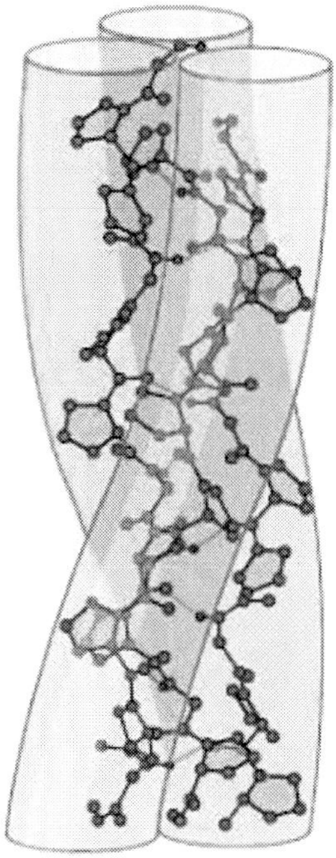

Figure 1. Collagen structure model.

Heterogeneous type I collagen, which possesses similar structural characters with human type I collagen, shows outstanding biocompatibility and potential bioactivity. The researches in the latest decade indicate that the heterogeneous type I collagen ideally performs in the field of biomedical researches and clinic applications. The versatile advantages of type I collagen make it one of the most favorable starting materials for biomaterials. At present, it is reported that the type I collagen-based biomaterials applied but not limited in drug delivery or cells carrier system, tissue engineering scaffold, surface modification etc. Although the researches are blooming and lots of achievements are reported, the quality of type I collagen is not seriously evaluated before the utilization. The composition and structure of collagen, which are the main features of the quality, will affect the behavior and performance of collagen-based biomaterials in a great degree. As a natural product, the collagen characterizations are primarily determined by the preparation methods, which have general similar processes but vary in details according to the different raw materials or application targets. In this chapter, the preparation processes of bovine type I collagen and the features of each preparation stage will be introduced. The characterization of collagen will be presented and the risk of collagen as the starting materials for tissue regenerative products will be discussed. Finally, the classification of type I collagen-based biomaterials will be reviewed according to recent advances on researches and applications, with focusing on the collagen-based hydrogels in cartilage defect reconstruction.

2. Preparation of Type I Collagen

The biosynthesis process of collagen is clearly understood and summarized in several literatures since 1960-70s [2-4]. Accordingly, type I collagen is fabricated *in vivo* after experiencing a long and complex process, from amino acids to fibers, from nanosize to bundles, from intracellular to extracellular. To obtain the type I collagen with ideal performance for biomedical purposes, the supreme preparation process should contain the gentle disassembly of collagen bundles and reverse the biosynthesis processes back to fibrillar collagen without non-helical telopeptides. Differed from the biosynthesis of collagen, which is driven by collaboration of enzymes and other bio-factors *in vivo*, the preparation of ideal collagen is complicated and difficult because of not only limited effects of chemicals and biological enzymes, but also the multifaceted compositions in animal tissues or organs, which might reduce or even eliminate the function of chemicals or enzymes used. Consequently, the pretreatment of the raw materials for collagen preparation is as important as the extraction process. In addition, the variety of sources requires a pretreatment to even the raw material conditions before moving to the next stage. Accordingly, combined with our research and experience on collagen preparation, we divide the preparation process into three stages: pretreatment stage, extraction stage and purification stage.

2.1. Pretreatment Stage

Calf skin and tendon contain a high proportion of native type I collagen, and thus are the main raw materials for bovine type I collagen. The collagen in the newborn calf skin has a high content of hydroxyproline, which is a feature amino acid in collagen. The research confirms that the hydroxyproline plays an important role in the construction and thermal stability of triple helix structure [5]. However, either skin or tendon has disadvantages. As the largest organ of animal body, the skin contains not only matrix networks but also cells, muscles, fats, blood and vessels and other appendages, such as the glands and hair follicles. Even in the matrix network, there are several different kinds of fibers, including collagen, elastic fibers. The non-collagen compositions in calf skin are complex and become an obstacle for collagen extraction. Meanwhile, there is a symbiosis of type I collagen with other collagen types, mainly type III collagen. On the other hand, the collagen content in tendon is higher than that in skin. But the collagen bundles in tendon are extremely tight and are enwrapped by basement membranes, which contain type IV collagen. Therefore, the pretreatment of raw materials before the extraction process is necessary to ensure a high yield of quality collagen product. Here, we take new born calf skin as typical raw material to introduce the pretreatment.

Granulating

The collagen fiber bundles in different areas of skin show distinguishing compactness. For example, the collagen network in butt is tighter than that in belly. Meanwhile, the whole piece of skin normally cannot be treated at one time. To reduce the differences between batches and influences of area differences, it is wise to cut or granulate the skin into pieces and regroup the pieces into different batches. Furthermore, with the enlarged superficial area, the granulated skin is helpful to raise the pretreatment and further extraction efficiency.

Unhairing

The skin is wholly covered with hairs, which should be removed early in the pretreatment. The incomplete removing hair or hair segments in the raw material need a high cost to clean out in the following process. In general, the hairs can be removed by mechanical shaving or chemicals. The hand-shaving will have no influence on the native collagen, but the efficiency is low and the hair roots are not easy to be removed. The chemical unhairing can eliminate the hair and roots effectively, but the strong alkaline environment possibly destructures the intact collagen during the process. In addition, the epidermis of the skin will be removed during the unhairing as well. Therefore, the efficiency and quality of collagen should be actually considered.

Degreasing

The fat or grease is extensively existent in animal tissues. The subcutaneous fat can be handily removed, but the removing of grease has to depend on the chemicals. Generally, the degreasing agent prepared by mixing of trichloromethane and ethanol is applied. The surfactants such as sodium dodecylsulphate (SDS) are utilized in some cases. Except the possible effect on the structure of protein, the worries on the remaining of chemicals, which have significant influence to the biocompatibility of products, exist for a long period.

Removing of Heavy Metals

There are several reasons leading to the skin containing heavy metals, such as lead, mercury, tin, silver, copper and so on. The heavy metals may exist in fodder or water, and gradually accumulate in the skin. In the pretreatment process, ethylene diamine tetraacetic acid (EDTA) is frequently used to couple the metals. And the repeating use of EDTA solution can increase the removing efficiency.

2.2. Extraction Stage

With the pretreatment of the calf skin, the collagen network is relatively pure and ready for the extraction treatment. Generally, there are three methods to obtain collagen, that is, neutral salting, acid dissolving, and enzyme digestion. In the collagen matrix, there is few uncross-linked collagen, which is free in the network and will be salting in the solution when the electrolyte concentration is appropriate. Acid dissolving normally conducted by using diluted hydrochloric acid or acetic acid. The acid will collapse the collagen network by breaking down the peptide linkage randomly. The separated collagen segments and the uncross-linked collagen chain will be dissolved in the acid solution and then be extracted. Both neutral salting and acid dissolving methods possess the shortcomings, including low yield and broad distribution of collagen segments. In comparison, the enzyme digestion method can acquire high yield of collagen with controlled molecular weight distribution. And more importantly, the specific enzyme (for example, pepsin) can digest at the target sites of the collagen chain, which will break down the network and remove the non-helical segments from the chain. The non-helical segments, which are located at the ends (carboxyl terminal and amino terminal) of collagen chain respectively, are the main source leading to immunological response of heterogeneous biomaterials. Therefore, the removing of non-helical domains from collagen will improve the quality of the collagen and further reduce the adverse reactions after implanting *in vivo*. In general, pepsin is the most widely applied enzyme in collagen extraction stage. Pepsin will cleave the specific peptide bond at the Tyr, which is existed at the both end of the helical chain. Concretely, the Tyr (Y) residues exist at 165, 167, 1195, 1214 and 1215 of bovine type I collagen's amino acid sequence listed in Figure 2. In addition, pepsin has the best activity under the acidic condition. Usually, pepsin is utilized with a certain concentration of acetic acid, which is helpful to loosen the collagen bundles or network. Consequently, the pretreated raw material digested by pepsin in acidic condition at 4°C is the most suitable and effective method to extract collagen for biomedical application.

Table 1. The segments in bovine collagen α-1(1) chain

Feature key	Position(s)	Length	Description
Signal peptide	1-22	22	
Propeptide	23-161	139	N-terminal propeptide
Helical chain	162-1215	1054	Collagen α-1(1) chain
Propeptide	1216-1463	248	C-terminal propeptide

The sequence in dash line frame is signal peptide (1-22) and the sequences in solid line frame are N-terminal (23-161) and C-terminal (1216-1463) propeptide, respectively. The sequence between 161 and 1215 is the helical chain segment.

The routine of collagen extraction by pepsin goes as follows. The pretreated skin is soaked in 0.5 M acetic acid with a liquor ratio higher than 40, based on the dry weight of the skin (the same hereinafter). The pH of the solution is around 2.5. Then, the 1-3 wt% pepsin powder is carefully weighed and added into the above solution after it is dissolved in a little 0.5 M acetic acid. The digestion process holds for 1-6 days with/without agitation. The viscosity of the pepsin-digested solution increases with the time expending. To stop the digestion, the enzyme is deactivated by temporary adjusting the solution pH to alkalescency (pH 7.5-9.0) and holding for 4-12 hours. After the digestion process, the collagen-containing solution can be attained by centrifugation of the pepsin-digested mixture. Commonly, high speed refrigerated centrifuge is necessary to ensure the separation efficiency and intact collagen structure. Then, the obtained supernatant is neutralized by NaOH solution. The collagen can be precipitated by adding neutral salts. Several kinds of neutral salts can be served as the salting agent. One of the most common salts is sodium chloride. Subsequently, the granulated dry sodium chloride is weighed and gently added into the clear solution under stirring, to a final concentration of 20-25 wt% or 3.0-4.0 mol/L (take NaCl for instance). After the completely dissolve of salt, the collagen-containing mixture is held statically for 8-12 hours to have the collagen fully precipitated. Following the centrifugation of the solid-liquid mixing solution, the precipitation is collected as crude collagen. Finally, the crude collagen is dissolved in 0.5 M acetic acid to further purification. The whole extraction process is conducted at 4 °C.

```
MFSFVDLRLL LLLAATALLT HGQEEGQEEG QEEDIPPVTC VQNGLRYHDR DVWKPVPCQI    60
CVCDNGNVLC DDVICDELKD CPNAKVPTDE CCPVCPEGQE SPTDQETTGV EGPKGDTGPR   120
GPRGPAGPPG RDGIPGQPGL PGPPGPPGPP GPPGLGGNFA PQLSYGYDEK STGISVPGPM   180
GPSGPRGLPG PPGAPGPQGF QGPPGEPGEP GASGPMGPRG PPGPPGKNGD DGEAGKPGRP   240
GERGPPGPQG ARGLPGTAGL PGMKGHRGFS GLDGAKGDAG PAGPKGEPGS PGENGAPGQM   300
GPRGLPGERG RPGAPGPAGA RGNDGATGAA GPPGPTGPAG PPGFPGAVGA KGEGGPQGPR   360
GSEGPQGVRG EPGPPGPAGA AGPAGNPGAD GQPGAKGANG APGIAGAPGF PGARGPSGPQ   420
GPSGPPGPKG NSGEPGAPGS KGDTGAKGEP GPTGIQGPPG PAGEEGKRGA RGEPGPAGLP   480
GPPGERGGPG SRGFPGADGV AGPKGPAGER GAPGPAGPKG SPGEAGRPGE AGLPGAKGLT   540
GSPGSPGPDG KTGPPGPAGQ DGRPGPPGPP GARGQAGVMG FPGPKGAAGE PGKAGERGVP   600
GPPGAVGPAG KDGEAGAQGP PGPAGPAGER GEQGPAGSPG FQGLPGPAGP PGEAGKPGEQ   660
GVPGDLGAPG PSGARGERGF PGERGVQGPP GPAGPRGANG APGNDGAKGD AGAPGAPGSQ   720
GAPGLQGMPG ERGAAGLPGP KGDRGDAGPK GADGAPGKDG VRGLTGPIGP PGPAGAPGDK   780
GEAGPSGPAG PTGARGAPGD RGEPGPPGPA GFAGPPGADG QPGAKGEPGD AGAKGDAGPP   840
GPAGPAGPPG PIGNVGAPGP KGARGSAGPP GATGFPGAAG RVGPPGPSGN AGPPGPPGPA   900
GKEGSKGPRG ETGPAGRPGE VGPPGPPGPA GEKGAPGADG PAGAPGTPGP QGIAGQRGVV   960
GLPGQRGERG FPGLPGPSGE PGKQGPSGAS GERGPPGPMG PPGLAGPPGE SGREGAPGAE  1020
GSPGRDGSPG AKGDRGETGP AGPPGAPGAP GAPGPVGPAG KSGDRGETGP AGPAGPIGPV  1080
GARGPAGPQG PRGDKGETGE QGDRGIKGHR GFSGLQGPPG PPGSPGEQGP SGASGPAGPR  1140
GPPGSAGSPG KDGLNGLPGP IGPPGPRGRT GDAGPAGPPG PPGPPGPPGP PSGGYDLSFL  1200
PQPPQEKAHD GGRYYRADDA NVVRDRDLEV DTTLKSLSQQ IENIRSPEGS RKNPARTCRD  1260
LKMCHSDWKS GEYWIDPNQG CNLDAIKVFC NMETGETCVY PTQPSVAQKN WYISKNPKEK  1320
RHVWYGESMT GGFQFEYGGQ GSDPADVAIQ LTFLRLMSTE ASQNITYHCK NSVAYMDQQT  1380
GNLKKALLLQ GSNEIEIRAE GNSRFTYSVT YDGCTSHTGA WGKTVIEYKT TKTSRLPIID  1440
VAPLDVGAPD QEFGFDVGPA CFL                                          1463
```

Figure 2. The whole sequence of bovine collagen α-1(1) chain (from UniProtDB, P02453 [6]).

During the extraction process, there are several frequently encountered problems. For example, the digestion duration varies in the literature. In some cases, the digestion lasts for less than 24 hours when the skin is homogenized and kept on stirring during the process. While in some other cases, the digestion duration is as long as 6-7 days in the condition of portioned skin and statical environment. Thus, the question is how to judge and decide the finishing point of digestion, and why? According to our research, the finishing point of digestion is relative to at least two aspects. Firstly, the viscosity of the system can be one of the indexes of the finishing point. It is obviously that the viscosity of the solution increases when the digestion proceeds. That is, more of pepsin-digested collagen dissolved in the acidic medium. In the high viscosity solution, the chance of interaction between enzyme and its substrate decreases and the rate of mass transfer declines sharply as well. Consequently, the extraction efficiency is sliding fast when the system viscosity is high, and the digestion process can be terminated when the viscosity climbs to a certain value.

Secondly, the activity of enzyme gradually attenuates during the digestion, especially when the pH is around 2.5, which is the optimum condition to pepsin. We carried out a research on the enzyme kinetics in the pepsin-digesting collagen extraction process. Small granules of calf skin were used, the ratio of acidic solution to the weight of raw materials is 40 and the whole digestion process is under agitating. A small amount of digested collagen-containing solution is sampled to test the content of hydroxyproline at different intervals. The variation trend of hydroxyproline contents can be considered as the collagen extraction rate and further calculated as the rate of the enzyme reaction. Also, the rate of the enzyme reaction can be described by Michaelis-Menten equation, which expresses the relationship between digestion rate and substrate concentration and shown as follows.

$$v = \frac{V_{max} \cdot [S]}{K_m + [S]}$$

The results of hydroxyproline contents at different intervals are shown as the symbols in the figure 3(a). And the process can be mathematically simulated by Michaelis-Menten equation shown as the line in the figure 3(a). The results indicate that the equation can fit the process very well with adj. R-square of 0.9876. To better understand the change of enzyme reaction rates, the derivative curve is made on the basis of simulation equation. From the curves, we can find that the enzyme react quickly at the initial period which lasts for less than 10 hours, and then reach a relative stable situation after around 20 hours. The results are consistent with the phenomena observed in the digestion process and our understandings. Therefore, the better efficiency might be achieved by limited digestion duration and add the pepsin gradually to maintain the enzyme activity at a high level in the system.

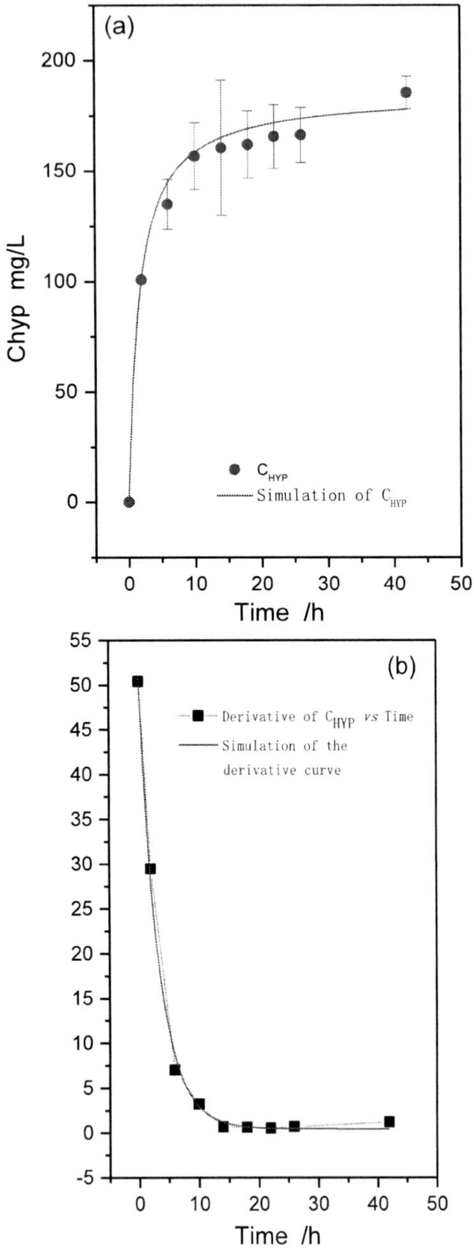

Figure 3. The hydroxyproline contents and the simulation curves during the extraction process.

2.3. Purification Stage

The collected crude collagen in the extraction stage includes collagen, neutral salts and non-collagen proteins. Necessary purification will remove the impurities in crude collagen; also it will narrow down the molecular weight distribution of collagen. Conventionally, repeat dissolving and gradient salting out is an effective and easy way to eliminate most of the unwanted non-collagen proteins. According to our research, the preliminary purification process can be optimized guided by Cohn "salting out" equation.

$$lgS=\beta-K_s\mu$$

where S is the protein solubility constant (g/L); μ is the ion activity; β and K_s are constants characteristic of the particular ion. β is independent of the salt but affected by temperature, solution pH and protein type; while K_s is connected with the salt and protein type but not decided by temperature and solution pH. According to Cohn's equation, the salting out methods can be divided as K_s type and β type. The K_s type means keeping the temperature and pH as constant but changing the ionic strength. The β type is making the ionic strength fixed and changing the pH and temperature. Since the proteins are sensitive to the ionic strength, K_s type salting out normally applied in collagen extraction stage to avoid coprecipitation of protein. The β type salting out can be used in the purification of collagen owing to that the solubility of collagen is relatively small and stable under certain condition, leading to a high resolution of precipitation.

The routine of collagen purification is dissolving the crude collagen in 0.5 M acetic acid firstly. Since the k_s type salting out is applied in the collagen extraction stage, the β type salting out is beneficial to the purification process. The weighed neutral salt is added into the re-dissolved collagen solution under gentle stirring. After the fully dissolving of the salt, the pH of the solution is adjusted to 7.0 by NaOH solution. Following the statically preserve for 4-12 hours, the collagen can be collected by high speed centrifugation. Then, the collagen can be dissolved again to have another round of salting out. Two or three rounds of dissolving and K_s and/or β methods salting out can purify the collagen at a large extent.

The collagen underwent repeat dissolving and K_s or β salting out contains a large number of salt. Dialysis is the easiest method to remove the salt. The precipitated collagen is loaded into the dialysis bags and dialyzes against abundant deionized water or acidic solution. Frequent change of the dialysate and stirring will accelerate the migration of ions. In general, it will take 4 to 10 days to remove the salts from the collagen. Alternative methods of desalination include size exclusion chromatography, ultrafiltration and so on. But these methods have disadvantages such as inadequate treatment capacity, the limited efficiency and need many consumables, resulting in a rare application based on the cost consideration.

The question concerned during the collagen preparation is what kind of neutral salt should be applied? Hofmeister series or lyotropic series can be the guideline of salting agents. The series is a classification of ions in order of their ability to salt out or salt in proteins. Anions appear to have a larger effect than cations, and partial of them are usually ordered as: $F^- \approx SO_4^{2-} > HPO_4^{2-} > CHCOO^- > Cl^- > NO_3^- > Br^- > ClO_3^- > I^- > ClO_4^- > SCN^-$. The order of cations is usually given as: $NH_4^+ > K^+ > Na^+ > Li^+ > Mg^{2+} > Ca^{2+}$. Therefore, a neutral salt combined by anion and cation, which are in the front of the orders, has strong ability to salt out the collagen from the solution. Ammonium sulfate and sodium chloride are the most frequently used salts to precipitate the protein, and the former has an even stronger precipitation effect. However, the biomedical product has strict requirements on salt type and content, leading to the limit application of ammonium sulfate.

Another issue being discussed is the desalinate efficiency. The dialysis process is easy to handle and effective to remove the salt in collagen solution. However, lots of traditional dialysis bags are of very limited capacity. In addition, the dialysis duration is so long that it almost accounts for half of the production cycle. Hence, the desalination treatment, particularly the dialysis process is the bottleneck of the production efficiency.

3. Characterization of Type I Collagen

The superiority of collagen as the starting material for biomedical applications is derived from manifold essential characteristics, which is decided by the preparation method and will affect the application performance. The International Organization for Standardization (ISO), American Society for Testing and Materials (ASTM), CEN/CENELEC and standard organization in other countries have issued equivalent or similar guidelines to regular the medical products. But there has no specific standard issued on collagen or collagen-based biomaterials with specific pass/fail criteria due to the variant forms of collagen products. As a natural polymer with specific characteristics, the composition of collagen is easily contaminated and the structure is vulnerable to physical, chemical and biological effect. Any unwanted or unexpected change on the composition or structure of collagen will lead to the partial or full disablement of the final functions. Although the characterization of collagen is important, numerous studies consider nothing or little about if the collagen met the requirements for the research of collagen-based biomaterials. To achieve consensus conclusions on collagen-based biomaterials, it is necessary to establish an effective, operative and commonly accepted standard to normalize the collagen as the starting material for biomedical uses. However, understanding what and how to characterize collagen product should enjoy the priority. The characterization of collagen can be evaluated from four aspects, including the composition analysis, structure characterization, performance assessment and biocompatibility evaluation.

3.1. Composition Analysis

As a form of a polypeptide chain, the amino acid sequence of collagen is defined as the primary structure. The composition of type I collagen is determined by the primary structure, and there are few interspecies differences in the primary structure of type I collagen. However, according to the preparation method, the composition of collagen might vary due to the remains of non-collagen protein, impurity substance, and partially degraded collagen. The composition analysis is essential in the standard of collagen, but it is not easy to understand all the composition quantitatively. On the other hand, no matter qualitative or quantitative analysis of the composition, it is not truthful to assure the test samples are type I collagen according to the results. But can only judge the samples' similarity to the features of type I collagen.

Water Content

It is an index specially employed to solid collagen products, including films, membranes, sponges and scaffolds. Since the collagen structure is sensitive to heat, the water in collagen products cannot be easily and entirely removed. Lyophilization is one of the most operative methods to remove the moisture in collagen products. However, water exists in almost all forms of dry collagen products. A typical lyophilizated collagen sponge or scaffold has moisture content around 5-10%. The water itself in collagen has no obvious influence to the collagen quality, but it may affect the quality and shelf life of the products if the products are sterilized by gamma radiation. Destructive examination like thermogravimetric analysis can determine the water content in collagen samples.

Solid Content

It is an index defined to collagen solution or hydrogels. For collagen solution, the solid content is equal to protein content. For collagen hydrogels, the solid content may higher than protein content since there are buffer reagents, neutralization reagents in the product. The results of solid content can be calculated by subtracting the water content.

Protein Content

As a special kind of protein, collagen and other possible included protein in collagen product can be measured by classical protein detection methods, such as Kjeldahl determination, Lowry (Folin-phenol) methods, Biuret test, and bicinchoninic acid (BCA) Protein Assay. Generally, Kjeldahl determination can be applied no matter collagen product is solid or liquid, and the accuracy is excellent and the interference factor is less (unless ammonium salt is utilized as the neutral salt). Other spectrophotometry can only apply to liquid collagen samples.

Purity

The purity should be defined as the collagen content in the product, which often be confused with protein content. As mentioned above, non-collagen protein and collagen segments or fractions may be included in the products, thus the content of collagen or purity differs from the protein content. At present, there is no method to directly measure the content of collagen. The widely accept method to determine the purity is a semi-quantitative measurement by sodium dodecyl sulfate polyacrylamide gel electrophoresis (SDS-PAGE). Briefly, the detection goes as follows. The dyeing limit (Dl, the lowest protein quantity that can be detected) is determined by using a concentration gradient of bovine serum albumin (BSA) solution as a protein model in SDS-PAGE. The collagen sample can be prepared by dissolving the solid product or diluting the liquid product. The solid or liquid collagen product is completely degraded by type I collagenase to obtain enzyme-degraded collagen sample, which has the same concentration with the collagen sample. Then, the collagen sample (A), enzyme-degraded collagen sample (B), collagenase solution (C), BSA solution with a quantity of dyeing limit (D) and protein marker (E) are all loaded to run the SDS - PAGE test. Following the dyeing by coomassie brilliant blue, the gel is imaged and the band densities

(%) of the samples calculated. The results are marked as A, B, C, D and E, respectively. If the band density of enzyme-degraded collagen sample differ from that of collagenase solution, the purity (%) = A-(B-C). If there is no difference between B and C, the purity (%) ≥ 100%-Dl/(v*C_0), where Dl is the dyeing limit (μg), Dl is the loading volume (μL) and C_0 is the collagen concentration of the loading sample.

Amino Acid Analysis

Having a particular primary structure, the range and content of amino acids have distinguishing features in type I collagen. Since the general sequence Gly-X-Y, where proline often occupys X and hydroxyproline in the Y position, repeating in the type I collagen, the content of glycine is nearly one third of all the amino acids. Also, type I collagen is high in L-alanine (~10%), L-proline (~12%) and 4-hydroxyproline (~8%), low in sulfur and contains no L-tryptophan. Meanwhile, hydroxyproline and hydroxylysine are the distinctive amino acids in type I collagen. Routinely, amino acid analysis is performed by full-automatic amino acid analyzer, with the hydrolyzed collagen.

Hydroxyproline Content

As the distinguish amino acid in type I collagen, hydroxyproline plays an important role in the maintaining of the triple helix structure. The intramolecular hydrogen bonds formed by hydroxyproline are vital to the stability of collagen structure, especially the thermal stability [5]. The dysfunction of hydroxylation of proline is one of the major reasons results in some collagen disables. The hydroxyproline content of type I collagen varies from 8% to 14% depending on the animal age and areas of calf skin. Normally, the hydroxyproline content is high in newborn or young calf skin, and decreases with the animal growth. Excepted the amino acid analysis mentioned above, the hydroxyproline content can be measured by spectrophotography after the completely hydrolyzed collagen solution being oxidized by chloramine-T and chromogenic reaction with paradimethylaminobenzaldehyde.

Impurity Contents

Any extraneous substances or materials in collagen can be classified as impurities, as described in ASTM F2212 [7]. The major impurities of concern include, but are not limited to the following: endotoxins, glycosaminoglycans (GAG), elastin, lipids, improperly aligned collagen molecules, host cell contaminants, cell culture contaminants, heavy metals, bioburden, viruses and chemical remains. At minimum, any protein impurity greater than 1% in the final collagen product should be identified and quantified. Even the presence of some impurities may have no adverse effect on product quality, their levels should be evaluated and controlled for lot-to-lot consistency. As ubiquitous in nature, endotoxin is one of the most difficult contaminations to be prevented. Endotoxin is stable and small enough to get through sterilizing filters. And the amount of endotoxin, which is critical to the product application, should be qualitatively measured for each new lot of collagen product. The endotoxin level should under regulatory limits to be allowed for human implantation. Mostly, the endotoxin content is determined by the gel clot test, which is the simplest and easiest of the Limulus amebocyte lysate (LAL) test methods. Carbohydrate content can be analyzed by classical gas-liquid chromatographic methods or spectrophotometric methods. Elastin can be tested by Western blots or ELISAs assay.

Heavy Metal Content

The heavy metal content usually separately evaluated to demonstrate it does not exceed a limit in the product specification. The heavy metals mentioned in the pretreatment stage of the collagen preparation are responding to the qualitative test method, which can be found in both Chinese Pharmacopeia and United States Pharmacopeia.

3.2. Structure Characterization

The natural triple-helix structure, which is considered as secondary structure, is vitally important to the characteristics of collagen. The collagen performance, including the thermal stability, mechanical strength, and the ability to engage in specific interactions with cells or other biomolecules (which is understood as bioactivity) is closely relative to the reservation of the structure.

Except the secondary structure of collagen molecules (or tropocollagen), the structure (superstructure) that they form collagen microfibril is deserved to be investigated. The collagen molecules can self-assemble into collagen microfibril under certain condition. This self-assembly process increases the size and complexity of collagen, and generates the macromolecular fibers which are essential components of tissue and organs *in vivo [5]*. In the biomedical study *in vitro*, the self-assembly is crucial to produce biomimetic extracellular matrix to hold cells and create an ideal microenvironment. Therefore, the appropriate characterization of collagen structure and superstructure is necessary to be included in the collagen standard when applied as biomedical material. In addition, comprehending the structural features of collagen is beneficial to the understanding of collagen stability and collagen-cell interactions.

Differential Scanning Calorimetry (DSC)

The triple helix structure of collagen will collapse or deform when collagen is heated, resulting in the denaturation of collagen. This thermal denaturation characteristic can be evaluated by DSC. This measurement not only detects the dissociation temperature of fibrils/microfibrils and denature temperature of collagen, but also reflects the crosslinking density in some collagen products. According to the literature, the onset of the transition temperature of intact collagen ranges from 39 °C to 64 °C [8, 9].

Circular Dichroism Spectra (CD)

CD is the most commonly used methods to study the secondary structure of proteins. The CD spectra in the far UV region (180 nm -240 nm) mostly probe the secondary structure of proteins, while the spectra in the near UV region (~240 nm -~350) monitors the side chain tertiary structures and microenvironment of aromatic amino acid residues. Since the secondary structure of collagen is distinguished left hand triple helix, which differs from that of common protein, the CD spectra of collagen have opposite peaks compared with the proteins having alpha structure. In general, the CD spectra of intact collagen have a positive peak at around 225 nm and a large negative peak at around 197 nm [10, 11].

Transmission Electron Microscopy (TEM)

Characterized with 1/4-stagger arrangement, native or self-assembled collagen fibers have a fibrillar period (D-period) around 67 nm with a gap/overlap structure, shown as figure 4. TEM is helpful in illustrating this structure information of collagen fibers or collagen superstructure. One of the most significant recent advances in collagen structure by TEM is the cryo-TEM techniques [12], which prepare 100 nm thick sections by cryosectioning and performing cryo-TEM at approximately -179 °C. Based on the image processing and averaging, the fibril periodicity of collagen can be clearly observed and measured.

Other methods to assist characterization of collagen are reported, including Atomic Force Microscope (AFM), Fourier Transform Infrared Spectroscopy (FTIR), etc.

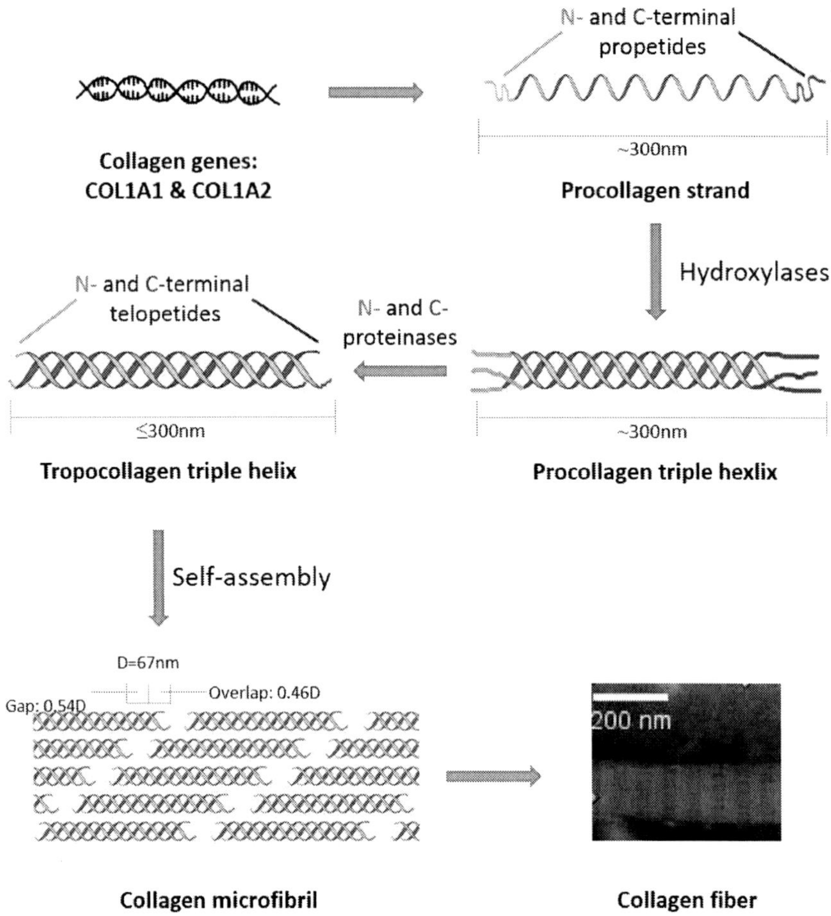

Figure 4. Biosynthetic route and the structure scheme of collagen fibers.

3.3. Performance Assessment

Excluded in the composition analysis and structural characterization of collagen, there are several properties which are affected by the preparation method and have obvious influences on the final functions of collagen-based biomaterials. These properties can be summarized as comprehensive performance of collagen, because they are decided not only by the compositions but also the conformations and fiber alignments. Briefly, the comprehensive performance includes mechanical strength, molecular weight and distribution, viscosity, isoelectric point, morphology, etc.

Molecular Weight and Distribution

Since type I collagen is derived from the COL1A1 and COL1A2 genes, the complete collagen chain which is associated by three alpha sub-chains has a molecular weight around 300 kDa. However, the molecular weight of the collagen will decrease and the distribution will be wide if the chain is cut during the preparation. SDS-PAGE is a convenient method to detect the molecular weight and distribution of collagen. The brief detection steps of SDS-PAGE have been introduced in the purity test in 3.1. With the bands of collagen and protein markers, the molecular weight can be calculated according to the following equation: $\lg M_r = \mathrm{k} - \mathrm{b}m_r$ where M_r is the molecular weight, m_r is the mobility ratio, which means the migration distance proportion of the band to the frontier, k and b are constants. In addition, the molecular weight distribution can be illustrated by SDS-PAGE at the same time.

Viscosity

The dissolved collagen molecule can be considered as a polypeptide, which is a special polymer distributed in solution. Therefore, the rheological knowledge of polymers can also apply in collagen study. Intrinsic viscosity is a molecular parameter which can be interpreted by the characteristics and conformation of the molecule, such as molecular weight, volume, shape, surface charge, deformation facility and so on. Intrinsic viscosity measurement is an economical and easy determination that yields useful information, although the resolution is limited and influence factors are numerous. According to the rheological theory, the intrinsic viscosity is related to the length-diameter ratio and the dispersion situation of collagen chains. The viscosity of acid-soluble collagen can be studied by rotational viscometry and capillary viscometry. For example, the intrinsic viscosity of a type I collagen sample we prepared is shown in figure 5. The viscosity study of collagen can reflect the structure and the measurement process, and is appropriate to be used to control the product quality in the industry. In addition, the viscosity can be a quality control or stability indicating parameter, which is relevant to the functionality of collagen and might be changed during the shelf life since the storage conditions are strict to some kinds of collagen products.

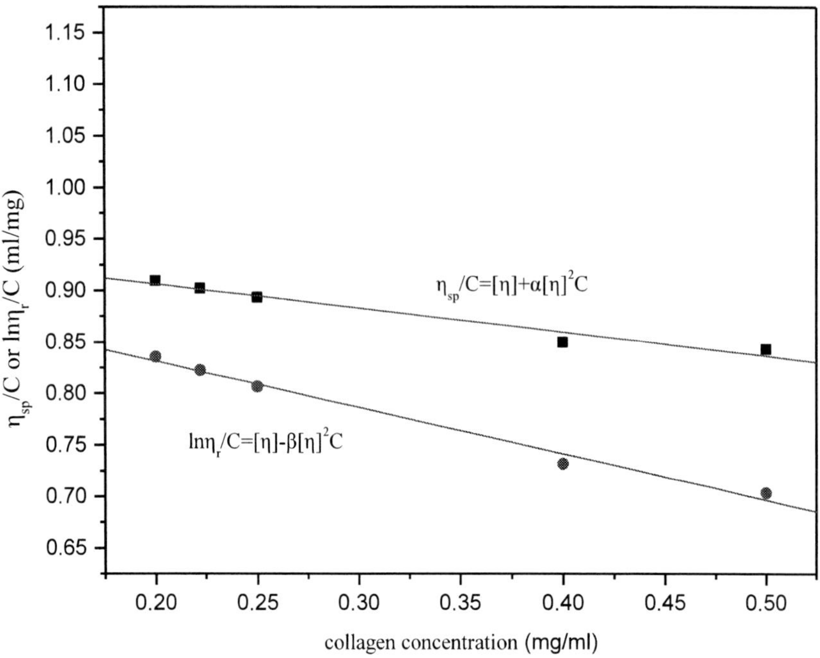

Figure 5. The extrapolation curve of collagen solution's viscosity.

Isoelectric Point (PI)

It is possible that the surface charge of collagen chain is positive or negative, because of both acidic and basic side groups exist in the molecule. The acid and enzyme used in the preparation process will break the polypeptide bundles at different sites, leading to exposure of different functional groups. The proportion of negative and positive groups determines the overall charge of collagen. Therefore, the PI of collagen can also reflect the performance of prepared collagen. Since the isoelectric point is defined as the pH at which the molecule carries no net electrical charge, the PI of collagen can be determined by neutralization of collagen solution and monitoring the zeta potential. A typical zeta potential curve of acid dissolving collagen neutralization process is shown in figure 6.

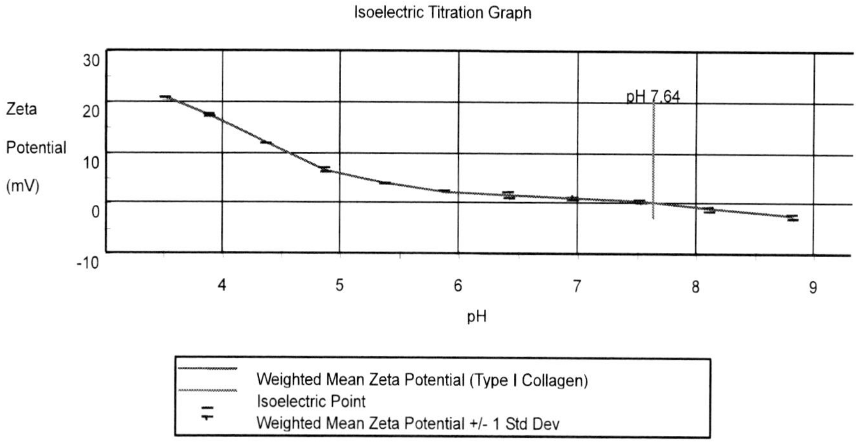

Figure 6. The zeta potential curve of neutralizing collagen solution.

3.4. Biocompatibility Evaluation

Biocompatibility, as well as immunogenicity, is one of the most concerned performances of collagen products. Although the type I collagen obtained from different animal species has extensive similarity in primary and higher order structure, the biocompatibility evaluation is required before the collagen-based biomaterials are applied for clinic applications. As the starting material for medical products, type I collagen should experience the same biocompatibility evaluations as other medical substrate materials, especially when new application, or modification to the material or physical forms of the material are considered. ISO 10993 Biological evaluation of medical devices (part1: Evaluation and testing within a risk management process) [13] provides a framework to plan a biological evaluation. Also, ASTM F 2212 (Standard guide for characterization of type I collagen as starting material for surgical implants and substrates for tissue engineered medical products) [7] introduces the guidelines for biocompatibility and immunogenicity evaluation. For type I collagen or collagen-based biomaterials, which will be applied in human implantation, following evaluations should be considered.

Cytotoxicity

The cytotoxicity evaluation of collagen product follows the methods introduced in ISO 10993 (part 5: Tests for *in vitro* cytotoxicity) [14]. Direct or indirect contact method can be chosen according to the application objective and the situation of the production. The result of the evaluation should be a numerical grader no greater than 1, meaning the product is considered to have no cytotoxic effect.

Irritation and Skin Sensitization

Both irritation and skin sensitization tests of collagen product are guided by ISO 10993 (part 10: Tests for irritation and skin sensitization) [15]. Normally, animal intracutaneous (intradermal) reactivity test is used to evaluate the irritation of collagen production. The requirements of the test are met if the final test sample score is 1.0 or less. Murine Local Lymph Node Assay (LLNA) or Guinea pig maximization test (GPMT) is alternative to test the skin sensitization of collagen production. For instance, the collagen product will be considered negative if the final calculated Stimulation Index is less than 3.0, with the test of LLNA.

Acute and Subacute Systemic Toxicity

ISO 10993 (part 11: Tests for systemic toxicity) [16] addresses the evaluation of generalized systemic toxicity of the medical devices, including acute and subacute systemic toxicity. Repeated or continuous exposure of test sample lasting for 90 days in rodents is used to evaluate the subacute systemic toxicity of collagen product. The collagen product should show negative acute and subacute systemic toxicity.

Genotoxicity

The genotoxicity test follows the method described in ISO 10993 (part 3: Tests for genotoxicity, carcinogenicity, and reproductive toxicity) [17]. To evaluate the genotoxicity of collagen product, a test for gene mutations in bacteria (OECD 471), a test for clastogenicity in mammalian cells (OECD 473), and a test for gene mutations in mammalian cells (OECD 476) are preferred test methods combination. The test results should be all negative to meet the requirements.

Biodegradation

The biodegradation of collagen product should refer to ISO 10993 (part6: Tests for local effects after implantation) [18], (part 9: Framework for identification and quantification of potential degradation products) [19], and (part 13: Identification and quantification of degradation products from polymeric medical devices) [20]. Since collagen product is sort of degradable/resorbable material and the degradation time varies depending on the preparation, in general, the subcutaneous or intramuscular implantation for 12 weeks is accepted. Compared to the negative control sample, the test samples of collagen product should be evaluated less than a slight irritant to the tissue via subcutaneous implantation to meet the requirements. After implanting *in vivo* for 12 weeks, the collagen product samples should be completely degraded.

3.5. Safety Discussion and Risk Control

As an animal derived substrate material for biomedical uses, collagen and collagen-based biomaterials are fiercely argued on its safety for human implantation during the passing decade. To avoid the potential risk, the administration department in some countries restricts the approval of new collagen-based biomaterials or tissue engineering products. At present, several regulations are issued to strengthen the supervision. Except to the biocompatibility evaluations such as acute toxicology test, subacute toxicology test, hypersensitivity test, and genetic toxicology test that are guided by ISO 10993, there are several other issues are concerned about collagen safety. Herein, we introduce the issues of great contention on bovine type I collagen in the recent years.

Transmissible Spongiform Encephalopathy (TSE) Agent Inactivation

SE, also known as prion diseases, will affect the brain and nervous system of many animals, and also humans. Unlike other kinds of infectious disease, the infectious agent in TSE is known as a type of protein, called TSE agent or prion protein. Prions can be transmitted through contact with infected tissue, body fluids or contaminated medical instruments. More importantly, it cannot be rendered to non-infectious by normal sterilization procedures, such as boiling or irradiating. Animals or human may infect with TSE by ingestion of infected foodstuffs, or by blood transfusion. Especially, the cattle may be infected genetically. And a type of TSE called bovine spongiform encephalopathy (BSE) spread in cattle in an epidemic fashion in recent decades. Therefore, TSE agents or prion protein may be introduced into collagen product as a result of raw materials sourcing. For bovine type I collagen preparation, it is a basic criteria to consider for safe sourcing and the tissue collection procedures to assure the raw materials is unlikely to contain TSE infectivity. On the other hand, the detection of the protease resistant of the ubiquitous prion protein in a tissue is necessary to avoid using the raw materials contain the transmissible agent, although a negative test of the protease resistant prion alone may not be sufficient. Also, it is required not only the feeding environment and fodder should be ecological, but the virus detecting and genetic background should be also recorded and filed. Other relevant guidelines of source documentation are introduced in ASTM F 2212 as well [7].

Viral Clearance

Except for TSE agent or prion protein, there are many other known viral pathogens existing in the raw materials for collagen preparation. It is necessary to monitor the sources with carefully detection and effective treatment to eliminate the potential infectivity. In bovine type I collagen preparation, viral clearance method may include detergent treatment, low pH, chemical treatments, and filtration or other purification method. Bae etc. studied the validity to remove and/or inactivate known and potential viral contaminants during the manufacturing process of bovine type I collagen [21]. They concluded that the 70% ethanol treatment and pepsin digestion at pH 2.0 has a sufficient virus-reducing capacity to inactivate the virus to undetectable levels, including bovine herpes virus (BHV), bovine viral diarrhea virus (BVDV), bovine parainfluenza 3 virus (BPIV-3) and bovine parvovirus (BPV). However, all the harsh treatments including chemical and biological treatments may not ensure complete viral inactivation.

Sterilization Method and Effects of Sterilization on Collagen Product

Most of the tissue engineering medical products are requested to being sterilized by a valid sterilization method, such as gamma irradiation, electronbeam, autoclaving or ethylene oxide. Unfortunately, those sterilization methods are so powerful that they possibly degrade the polypeptide chains or destroy the structure of native collagen, or have potential chemical reactions with the active groups in collagen. In general, solid collagen products sterilized by gamma irradiation or ethylene oxide, including films, membranes, and sponges may have a significant change in mechanical properties. The liquid collagen products, mainly solution and hydrogels, sterilized by gamma irradiation may lead to viscosity change or architecture broken. And the collagen solution is normally too sticky to pass through the filter, and the collagen molecule weight and shape hinder the filtration too. However, the influence on the product effectiveness should be further evaluated since the application approaches and clinical indications are diverse. The influence of sterilization on collagen product or collagen-based biomaterials should be evaluated during the establishment of production lines. Consequently, most of collagen products and collagen-based biomaterials are prepared by aseptic processing steps, but not sterilizing the final products. Only several sorts of cross-linked or modified collagen products can endure an approved sterilization method. As a result, the sterilization method should be chosen by the effectiveness of sterilization and primarily dictated by the effect on the product effectiveness.

4. Application of Type I Collagen in Tissue Regeneration

As a major extracellular matrix component and structural protein in connective tissue of mammal and human body, collagen has a long history of research and application in biomedical field because of its particular characteristics and easy availability. The researches of type I collagen in tissue regeneration advanced significantly in recent decade, however, the successful clinical application is very limited owing to various obstacles existing between laboratory bench and clinical sickbed. In recent years, collagen and collagen-based biomaterials are still one of the most emphasized natural polymers in research and application. Collagen or collagen-based biomaterials contain almost every form of biomedical products, such as surface coatings, thin films, membranes, microspheres, sponges, hydrogels and other pattern of scaffolds. In addition, collagen or collagen-based biomaterials were found in tissue regeneration research and application of almost every kind of connective tissues, including bone [22, 23], cartilage [24], vascular tissue [25], skin [26-28], and others [29]. When the biomaterials applied in the tissue engineering, the microenvironment of cells can be assorted to two-dimensional (2D) or three-dimensional (3D). It is reported that the cells attached and proliferated in 3D biomaterials show better phenotype and functional expression [30]. Herein, the progress of collagen-based biomaterials will be introduced on the basis of the different microenvironment that the biomaterials provided, namely 2D or 3D collagen-based biomaterials. It should be noted that the review of collagen application is not limited to bovine, but all animal derived type I collagen.

4.1. 2D Collagen-based Biomaterials

Type I collagen extracted from calf skin have been used to establish traditionally 2D monolayer culture systems, which are applied to investigate the regulation of cellular differentiation and cellular production of extracellular matrix. Further, the application of collagen advances to the surface modification of biomaterials, to improve the biocompatibility of the substrate or enhance the interactions between cells and biomaterials. With the development of the fabrication methods, other forms of 2D collagen-based biomaterials are studied and applied, including the film, sheet, disc and membrane, etc.

Surface Modification/Coating

As a major extracellular matrix, collagen has multi-functions in human tissues and has been proven to improve the attachment for many cell lines. Not only the functional cells, but also the human embryonic stem cells (hESCs) and induced pluripotent stem cells (iPSCs) can adhere on collagen coating and further derive to mesenchymal stem cell (MSC), which successfully differentiated *in vitro* into three different lineages: osteogenic, chondrogenic and adipogenic [31]. Consequently, collagen is widely applied to the surface modification of medical production for implantation, especially the products made of metals or polymers, which are considered to be inert materials *in vivo*.

Collagen Coating on Metal Substrates

Alloys made of metals have a long history of clinical application in biomedical engineering, especially in bone regeneration. However, the deficiencies of metal substrates are obvious. Patients need to receive fast and reliable rehabilitation, which can be understood as increasing the rate of osseointegration and minimizing the time for healing. Even though some porous scaffolds are developed, the interfaces between metal substrate and tissue are not satisfied. A possible solution is coating the substrates with bioactive factors, and collagen is one of the most popular proteins. For example, titanium (Ti) based alloy is widely researched and achievements are made on oral and bone implants. Tu et al. obtained surface modified titanium by mineralized collagen coating by electrolytical deposition. The results indicated the coating is stable in simulated body fluid and had good cytocompatibility [32]. Lafisco et al. modified the Ti substrate with collagen nano-fibers by electrospinning to simulate the extracellular matrix, and studied the biological performance by culturing stem cells on the samples. They concluded that the collagen coated showed faster osteoblastic differentiation and more efficient deposition of mineralized matrix than those uncoated substrates [33]. Another strategy is coating the substrate with an organic-inorganic combination. Wang et al. reported a hydroxyapatite (HA) with or without collagen was electrochemically deposited on a titanium metal, and arrived at a conclusion that the HA-collagen modified titanium had higher bioactivity than traditional ones [34]. Besides, collagen is utilized to modify the surfaces of other metal or alloy substrates, including tantalum (Ta) [35] and magnesium (Mg) [36]. Also, researchers investigated the adhesion energy of type I collagen on smooth and rough ceramic rutile TiO_2 and α-Al_2O_3 by molecular dynamic simulations. They found that the adhesion to rutile TiO_2 surface is far stronger than that to the α-Al_2O_3 surface [37].

Collagen Coating on Polymer Substrates

The usually investigated synthetic polymers have advantages in high and controlled mechanical properties, biodegradability and various manufacturability, showing an expansive potential in tissue engineering. However, the polymer-based scaffolds have adverse conditions as well. For example, the polylactide (PLA), poly(lactide-co-glycolide) (PLGA) or polycaprolactone (PCL) is highly hydrophobic causing poor initial cell attachment and proliferation. Coating by collagen is an easy and effective way to improve on this weakness. Cai et al. develop a novel approach to fabricate a sequential alkali hydrolysis of PLA, which produce a density gradient of carboxyl group moieties onto the films, and then covalently linked with collagen. With these collagen surface-density gradients on PLA films, the endothelial cells show different behaviors [38]. Kiran et al. modified the surface of PCL and nano-hydroxyapatite scaffold to introduce free NH_2 groups, which enabled the immobilization of collagen to modulate cellular activity and biological functions [39]. Sugiyama et al. reported the cells were homogeneously throughout the collagen coated PLA sponge [40]. Yu et al. prepared PLGA microspheres and then coated with collagen to adhere bone mesenchymal stem cells. Three months after the materials injected into the intertrochanters of SD rats, the BMSCs seeded PLGA/Col microspheres promoted trabecular reconstruction and improved bone quality in osteoporotic rats [41]. Kawase et al. used poly(L-lactide-co-epsilon-caprolactone) film and modified the substrate with collagen[42]. Lee et al. coated the PCL/β-TCP scaffolds with collagen layer to improve the performance of the scaffolds [43]. They all drew the conclusion that the collagen coating modified the hydrophobic nature of the polymer and improved the initial cell adhesion and biological functions. With the development of electrospinning technology, nanofibrous PLA or PCL and further porous membranes or scaffolds are prepared. The collagen is utilized to improve the cell attachment of these products as well as it applied on dense polymer substrates. Chen et al. had collagen grafted on nanofibrous PLA membrane to improve the bioactivity for cartilage tissue engineering [44]. Hong et al. studied the preparation, physical properties and cellular activity of collagen coated electrospun PCL [45]. More researches with PLA and/or PCL fibers are reported and reach a similar conclusion [46-49]. Except for the PLA, PLGA and PCL, collagen coating is applied on other polymer to improve the performance or cryopreservation of cells, such as poly(3-hydroxybutyrate-co-3-hydroxyvalerate) (PHBV) [50, 51], polyurethane (PU) [52]and polyvinyl formal (PVF) [53].

Novel Coating or Evaluation Technology

The traditional surface modifications by collagen are achieved by physical adsorption, electrochemical deposition, or chemical cross-linking. Some novel methods to prepare collagen coating are reported in recent years. One of the advances is the pattern coating or oriented assembly of collagen on substrates, to control and trigger specific tissue response. Differ from the layer-by-layer multilayer assembly method [54], Thickett et al. produced a patterned polystyrene surface by dewetting of metastable poly(N-vinylpyrrolidone) (PNVP), and achieved micropattern of collagen by different adsorption conditions[55]. Stylianou et al. compared the fibroblasts morphology and alignment on collagen films consisted by randomly oriented and oriented collagen fibers, whose nanostructure can be controlled by formation methods. Their investigation is helpful to elucidate the mechanism of cell-biomaterials interactions and enable the design of intelligent coating for implants [56, 57]. Pastorino et al. reported another way to form oriented collagen nanocoating. They used Langmuir-Blodgett technique to form a stable collagen film at the air-water interface and the Langmuir-Schaefer deposition was adopted to transfer it to the support surface. The *in vitro* test with 3T3 cells showed great cells proliferation and alignment [58]. Bosco et al. applied electrospray deposition (ESD) to coat titanium disks with alkaline phosphatase and collagen at room temperature, and they found ESD was successful to deposit organic molecules preserving their properties [59].

Coating on Collagen Substrate

Collagen can be used not only as coating material, but also substrate too. Since the collagen scaffolds have outstanding properties, they are studied as substrate to improve the application performance via coated by other materials. Cooper et al. modified collagen modules by coating fibronectin to avoid the host inflammation and limited human umbilical vein endothelial cell (HUVEC) survival, which happened when pure collagen modules covered by HUVEC are subcutaneous implanted in immunocompromised mice [60]. Hirata et al. treated the collagen scaffolds by multiwalled carbon nanotubes, and evaluated the constructs by rat primary osteoblasts culture and tissue responses. The results indicated that the constructs contained significantly higher level of ALP, calcium and osteopontin than the uncoated scaffolds. Meanwhile, significantly more bone formation was observed around the constructs after implanted for 28 days [61]. Similar research was done by Baktur and Kim et al., [62, 63]. Differ from their research, Kanayama et al. applied other types of carbon, which are graphene oxide (GO) and reduced grapheme oxide (RGO). After implanted into subcutaneous tissue on the backs of rats, the RGO coated constructs shown effective for osteogenic differentiation than those of GO coated and uncoated constructs [64]. Yang et al. modified the collagen scaffolds with apatite coating to prolong the release rate and period of BMP-2, which was carried in the collagen scaffolds [65, 66].

Film/Membrane

As the most common forms of biomaterials, films or membranes have a long history of research and application, such as anti-adhesion film [67], corneal repair film [68], dermal substitute [69]. Collagen based films or membranes have a wide application in guided tissue regeneration, including the periodontal tissue regeneration, myocardial tissue engineering, skin tissue engineering and so on.

Application and Functionalization of Collagen Film/Membrane

Researches have conducted to compare the periodontal fibroblast spheroids response on collagen-based and synthetic membranes, and they had similar performance of cell proliferation and migration and the immunohistochemical properties [70, 71]. Koseoglu et al. treated Miller Class I gingival recession defect by collagen membrane with autologous gingival fibroblast and achieved a satisfied results [72]. In skin tissue engineering, Lammers et al. created a collagen membrane with a papillary structure, which mimicking the architecture of the human papillary dermis. Following the culture of primary human keratinocytes on the membranes, the microscopical, gene expression microarrays and immunohistochemical tests proven that the specific collagen architecture can direct keratinocyte behavior [73]. After understanding the properties of pure collagen membranes, researches tried to improve the performances or functions by different means. Taraballi et al. treated collagen films by plasma to functionalize the films surface with carboxyl and amino groups, and the films were improved for grafting bioactive molecules [74]. Liu et al. developed an antibacterial collagen film by loading tobramycin, and the physical, antibacterial properties and biocompatibility were characterized. The results were excellent after 3 months experiments [68, 75]. Calderon-Colon et al. improved collagen vitrigels for corneal reconstruction by increasing 11% in transmittance and 100% in tensile strength [76]. Forti et al. enhanced the properties and biocompatibility of collagen by using 1,4-Dioxane [77]. Gao et al. prepared collagen membranes loaded with human vascular endothelial growth factor (VEGF) fused by a specific peptide collagen-binding domain (CBD). The results of *in vivo* repairing the infracted myocardium in a rabbit model showed that the CBD-VEGF/collagen group had the effective penetration of cells and more vascularization in infarcted myocardium [78]. Yamano et al. compared the subsequent effects of the released platelet-derived growth factor (PDGF) and growth/differentiation factor 5 (GDF-5) from collagen membranes on bone regeneration *in vitro* and *in vivo* [79].

Composite Collagen-based Film/Membrane

There is a convenient way to overcome the weaknesses of collagen films is the preparation of composites by two or more components. Ho et al. dissolved polycaprolactone and collagen in 1,1,1,3,3,3-hexafluoro-2-propanol (HFP) to constitute the PCL-collagen blends, and prepared the meshes by electrospinning; the meshes are evaluated by mechanical tests and in vitro cell culture. The results supported the use of the mesh composed by 20% collagen as a cartilage patch [80]. He et al. conducted the similar research using poly(l-lactic acid-co-epsilon-caprolactone) (PCLC) and collagen with a sandwich construction model for cartilage regeneration [81, 82], while Liu et al. adopted polylactide-polyglycolide (PLGA) and collagen nanofibrous membranes for wound dressing [83]. Steele et al. prepared a collagen cellulose composite film and compared the mechanical properties, cells growth and histological performance against swine small intestine submucosa; the results indicated that the composite film was preponderant from all aspects [84].

Cross Linked Collagen-based Film/Membrane

Chemical cross linking is another effective method to improve the performance of collagen-based films. Traditionally, glutaraldehyde is applied as the cross linker of collagen films. Verissimo et al. improved the modification by progressive crosslinking, and studied the biocompatibility and degradation of collagen membranes [85]. Carbodiimide is one of the common cross linker since it is length-crosslinking. Grover et al. cross-linked collagen membranes with a carbodiimide and found a dramatic increase in the stiffness and also reduce the roughness of the films. Meanwhile, the crosslinking reduced the capacity to support cell activity and potentially limit the effectiveness of the collagen-based films [86]. Liu et al. fabricated a film with collagen, gelatin and hyaluronic acid by crosslinking with 1-ethyl-3-(3-dimethyl aminopropyl) carbodiimide (EDC) and N-hydroxysuccinimide (NHS), shown a potential use in cornea tissue engineering [87]. Li et al. prepared the collagen chitosan membrane by using the EDC as crosslinker and studied the optical transmittance of the membranes and discussed the potential application for corneal tissue engineering [88]. Wang et al. crosslinked collagen and chitosan by hot dehydrogenation firstly, and then secondary crosslinked chondroitin sulfate by Carbodiimide. The ternary membrane was applied as a wound dressing and achieved a good assessment [89]. Also, some other cross-linkers are applied to fabricate the collagen-based films or membranes. Sandri et al. used 1,4-butanediol diglycidyl ether (BDDGE) to crosslink collagen membrane and further tested and verified the possibility of application in cardiac tissue engineering [90]. Yamauchi et al. modified the collagen by 4-butyrothiolactone to obtain the mercapto group-bearing collagen, which had as high as 36MPa of tensile strength and was more resistant to the degradation by collagenase [91].

4.2. 3D Collagen-based Biomaterials

With the development of tissue engineering, researches realized that a three-dimensional scaffold would afford a better microenvironment for the cells, resulting in a better cell response including proliferation and phenotype expression etc. [30]. Cells niche, which is considered to be critical to the proliferation and differentiation of cells, is one of the most important aspects for the design and development of ideal scaffold in tissue engineering. Possessed the characteristic of biocompatibility and bioactivity, collagen is potential to fabricate the cells niche. Sponge and hydrogel are the most commonly studied 3D collagen-based biomaterials, which is the focus of the research in the recent years, although either sponge or hydrogel has almost insurmountable shortcomings. The development of collagen-based sponge and hydrogel in recent 5 years is reviewed.

Scaffold/Sponge

Due to the high similarity with extracellular matrix, collagen scaffold or sponge is extensively applied as one of the three elements of tissue engineering (cells, scaffolds and growth factors). Differ from the 2D film or membrane mentioned above, the collagen-based scaffold or sponge has an obvious porous architecture inside of the material. This feature of scaffold or sponge enables the cells to attach in a stereo microenvironment, which is closer to the native condition. Although it is considered that the cells attached in scaffold or sponge intrinsically proliferate in two-dimensional, the interactions between cells and materials are distinct from those on 2D films or membranes. Therefore, scaffold or sponge is considered as 2.5 dimensional biomaterials.

To fabricate the collagen-based scaffold or sponge suit for tissue engineering, type I collagen generally experiences various modifications or blends with other materials [92]. Among the diverse blended scaffolds or sponges, they can be classified according to the homogeneous or inhomogeneous distribution of the compositions or structure in unitary, binary, ternary or even quaternary materials. Herein, the collagen-based scaffold or sponge will be reviewed as unitary scaffold / sponge, homogeneous scaffold / sponge and inhomogeneous scaffold / sponge.

Unitary Scaffold/Sponge

There are two kinds of unitary collagen-based scaffold or sponge. Both of these two kinds of unitary scaffold or sponge have excellent progress in this decade. The first kind is the accellular collagen matrix, which is prepared by decellularization of animal or human tissues, such as accellular dermal matrix and accellular heart valve. The accellular collagen matrix remove all the cells and other substance that maybe results in immunological reaction after implantation, and have the advantages of elaborate structure which is close to nature human tissue. Strictly, the accellular matrix cannot be classified as collagen-based scaffold or sponge, but it still has a similar composition and structure. Tedder et al. prepared the fibrous scaffolds by decellularization of porcine pericardium and spongiosa, and further stabled the scaffolds on silicone molds by pentagalloyl glucose to create layered collagen constructs for heart valve tissue engineering [93].

Another kind of unitary collagen-based scaffold or sponge is prepared by dissolved collagen with or without cross linking. The important parameters of scaffold or sponge can be easily controlled or improved by the preparation techniques or modification. Chen's group fabricated funnel-like collagen sponge with open surface pore structure by freeze-drying method that used embossing ice particulates as a template. They investigated the size of ice particulates and freezing temperature [94], a gradient pore size structure [95] and the pore size effect on cartilage regeneration [96]. Khayyatan et al. carefully studied the influence of preparation parameters on the collagen scaffolds, and investigated the physical effects of collagen scaffolds on the behavior of human induced pluripotent stem cell (hiPSC) derived neural progenitors. The results suggested that the pore structure and laminin coating of collagen scaffolds significantly impact cell behavior [97]. Amruthwar et al. modified collagen scaffold with elastin-like polypeptides, and the results confirmed that the composites had increased physical and mechanical properties [98]. Monjo et al. developed collagen sponges loaded with rosuvastatin to enhance bone formation in critical-size cortical bone defects [99]. Since the collagen scaffolds exhibited significant levels of advanced glycation end products (AGES), Chow et al. treated the scaffolds with penta-galloyl glucose to reduce the scaffold-bound AGE levels and further mitigate the diabetes-related complications [100].

Spinning or electrospinning is an effective method to fabricate the collagen-based scaffold. Collagen fibers can be developed by spinning or electrospinning, and further fabricated the three dimensional mesh or scaffold to meet the requirements of tissue engineering. Carlisle et al. studied the mechanical stress-strain properties of single electrospun collagen nanofibers, and they found the small strain modulus of the nanofibers was 2.82GPa [101]. Burck et al. researched the structure of regenerated collagen nanofibers to answer the open question how much the spinning process preserves or alters the native structure of collagen. They concluded that the structure preservation was depending on the solvents and refolding was happened during the spinning process [102]. Nevertheless, Caves and Siriwardane et al. tried to prepare the collagen fibers by wet spinning technique, respectively. Cave et al. reported a continuous extrusion system to manufacture synthetic collagen fiber. With this system, collagen fibers with an ultimate tensile strength of 94MPa were produced at 60m/hr [103]. Siriwardane designed an automatic wet spinning device with precise control and utilized ammonium hydroxide and acetone as coagulation bath. The wet-spun collagen fiber had half a meter in length and further corsslinked by genipin, showing a benefit to dorsal root ganglion neurons and Schwanna cell survival and growth [104].

Homogeneous Scaffold/Sponge

Homogeneous scaffold or sponge is easy to be fabricated by blending the solutions and following drying. The composition or structure in the homogeneous scaffold or sponge is evenly distribution and isotropic, which means the uniform of performances and functions. The convenience of fabrication and operability encourages the research and application of collagen-based scaffold or sponge in the tissue engineering. Hempel et al. generated artificial extracellular matrices containing collagen and hyaluronan sulfate, and transforming growth factor beta 1 was adsorbed in the scaffold to promote the function expression of cultured human mesenchymal stromal cell [105]. Lloyd, et al. studied the influence and regulation of freezing rate to the structure of collagen-glycosaminoglycan scaffold by a controlled-rate freezing [106].

To enhance the tensile strength of collagen-based scaffold or sponge, lots of researches have been conducted to meet the demands for tissue engineering, especially bone tissue engineering. Shen et al. synthesized the hydroxyapatite (HAp) nano-particles and distributed homogeneously in collagen solution to fabricate homogeneous HAp/collagen nanocomposites. They found the mechanical performance was obviously increased [107]. Xia et al. fabricated a collagen-apatite scaffold with a unique multi-level lamellar structure consisting of co-aligned micro and macro pores, leading to a twelve-fold increase in Young's modulus and a two-fold increase in the compression modulus. Together with a good support of attachment and spreading of MC3T3-E1 osteoblasts, the constructs were considered to be applicable in bone regeneration [108]. Xiong et al. enhanced the strength of the porous collagen and hyaluronic composite scaffolds by adding bioactive nano-glass [109], while Hong et al. prepared bioactive glass fibrous filaments and embedded well within collagen network [110]. Zugravu, et al. prepared collagen-chitosan-calcium phosphate microparticle-based ternary scaffolds and compared the physical properties and cytocompatibility with scaffolds without collagen. The ternary scaffolds exhibited 0.6-1.2MPa Young's modulus, 23% degradation over 4 weeks and supported a 4-7 folds increase in osteoblast cell number over 7 days in culture [111].

Electrospinning is also applied to fabricate homogeneous blended fibers. Maghdouri-White et al. blended silk fibroin and collagen solution with different ratios, and prepared the fibers by electrospinning. The mechanical properties and cell response on the scaffold were studied [112]. Prabhakaran et al. fabricated both random and aligned composite poly(3-hydroxybutyrate-co-3- hydroxyvalerate) (PHBV) collagen nanofibers by electrospinning, and nerve cells were cultured on PHBV/collagen nanofibers to evaluate the potential for nerve regeneration. The results showed that the aligned PHBV/Col 50:50 nanofiber had the highest cell proliferation and appropriate cell morphology for nerve regeneration [113]. Similar composite polymer/collagen nanofiber were studied for nerve tissue engineering, including PLGA-silk fibroin-collagen [114], PLGA/collagen [115], PCL/collagen [116], P(LLA-CL)/collagen I/collagen III [117], and collagen/GAG [118] etc.

Inhomogeneous Scaffold/Sponge

The inhomogeneous scaffold or sponge is studied to highly mimetic the natural tissue or organ, where the compositions and structures are non-continuous distributed leading to a combination of diverse functions. The design and fabrication of inhomogeneous scaffold or sponge are mainly bio-inspired and aims to develop biomimic or smart constructs, which can response to the external simulations and meet the requirements better for the tissue regeneration. A particular pattern of inhomogeneous scaffold or sponge is a substrate scaffold or sponge embedded with microspheres, which are made by the same or different materials with the substrate. The microspheres can hold growth factors or some other proteins or drugs, which will release responding to the change of the environment. This delivery system loaded scaffold or sponge has an improved performance in tissue engineering than the traditional ones. Yu et al. prepared the gelatin microspheres incorporating basic fibroblast growth factor (bFGF), and embedded in collage sponge with different biodegradabilities. The *in vivo* tests of the constructs combined with human preadipocytes shown the regeneration of adipose tissue [119, 120]. On the other hand, Caliari et al. fabricated an inhomogeneous scaffold by another way. They created core shell collagen-glycosaminoglycan (CG) composites featured by integration of a low density, anisotropic CG scaffold core with a high density CG membrane shell. The tests indicated the composites maintained sufficient permeability and improved mechanical strength [121]. Tuzlakoglu et al. fabricated a nano- and microfiber combined scaffolds by electrospinning of collagen on starch-based fiber meshes, and further produced thicker constructs by layer-by-layer to meet the requirements of large bone defects [122].

Another type of inhomogeneous scaffold is trying to prepare the constructs with delicate structure, such as the transitional structure between the bone and the cartilage. Bian et al. fabricated the osteochondral β-TCP/collagen scaffold by ceramic stereolithography (CSL) and gel casting. A suitable binding force between cartilage phase and ceramic phase was achieved by physical locking [123].

Hydrogel

Similar with the compositions of human tissue, water is the main part of hydrogels. In some degree, the hydrous microenvironment fit the cells better than any other form of biomaterials [124]. The cells embedded in the hydrogels not only can attach to the architecture component of the hydrogels but also can proliferate in the stereo surroundings. The feature of hydrogel requires the cells involvement during the fabrication of hydrogels, while it is impossible for sponge to have cells planted during the preparation process. The cells introduction and culture methods are the major differences between hydrogel and scaffold. The fabrication parameters of collagen hydrogel and the properties most relevant for tissue engineering are studied and have been reviewed in literatures [124]. The hydrogels can be sorted as scaffolds introduced above, such as unitary hydrogels, homogeneous hydrogels and inhomogeneous hydrogels. However, the hydrogels are so versatile in tissue engineering and we prefer to review the collagen-based hydrogels by their clinical application.

Fabrication Improvement of Collagen-based Hydrogels

Since cells, especially bone marrow mesenchymal stem cells (MSCs), are sensitive to the surroundings, the preparation parameters of collagen hydrogels are carefully studied. To find the clues of controlling the differentiation fate of MSCs or matching the hydrogel properties with the environment of tissue defects, the preparation of collagen-based hydrogels are of great interest. Researchers should pursue strategies to modulate collagen hydrogel fibrillar density and organization in the mesostructure, to fabricate collagenous matrices with extracellular matrix-like features [125]. As one of the most distinct differences between native extracellular environment and collagen-based hydrogel, the density of collagen fibrils has great influence to the response of seeded cell. Abreu et al. discovered that the collagen density of hydrogels had significantly effect to the functional properties of scaffold, while a higher density would result in a higher storage modulus, platelet activation, fibroblast proliferation and scaffold retraction [126]. To date, there are mainly five strategies to modulate the fibrillar density in collagen hydrogel. Reverse dialysis: Knight et al. reported a reverse dialysis of collagen gels against 0.5% PEG to induce liquid crystallization [127]; Evaporation: collagen fibrillar ordered matrices were obtained by using the property of type I collagen monomers to self-assemble in liquid crystalline arrays by slow evaporation of acidic solutions at high concentrations, as Bessea et al. reported [128]; Plastic compression: Brown et al. introduced a process could rapid remove fluid from hyperhydrated collagen hydrogel using plastic compression, to produce dense, cellular and mechanically strong native collagen structures with controllable nano- and micro-scale biomimetic structures [129]; Continuous injection: Mosser et al. developed a protocol to produce dense organized collagen matrices by the organization of a collagen solution, which relied on the continuous injection into glass microchambers and then sol-gel transition [130]; and Gas aspiration-ejection (GAE): Marelli et al. introduced GAE, which was robust and simple method, to engineer three dimensional, anisotropic, cell seeded, injectable dense collagen hydrogels with controllable fibrillar densities, without using of crosslinking [125].

Collagen-based Hydrogels Applied as Wound Dressing and in Skin Tissue Engineering

The skin tissue engineering requires the hydrogels with excellent biocompatibility and moderate mechanical properties. Moreover, the wound dressing should have appropriate water adsorption capacity and water vapor permeability, which is especially beneficial to the wound regeneration. Therefore, the hydrogels applied in skin tissue engineering need architecture with interconnected and open pores. Wong et al. fabricated a pullulan-collagen composite hydrogels by a salt-induced phase inverse technique. The composite hydrogels shown excellent cytocompatibility *in vitro*, and the *in vivo* tests demonstrated improved wound closure with formation of vascularized granulation tissue [131]. Desimone et al. prepared hybrid and nanocomposites silica collagen based on concentrated collagen hydrogels, and evaluated *in vitro* and *in vivo*. The significantly improved mechanical and thermal stability and the satisfied in vivo results established the hydrogels potentialities for dressings [132]. To increase the mechanical stability of skin substitute to allow for safe and convenient surgical handling, Hartwell et al. created crosslinked collagen-GAG scaffolds containing polyvinyl alcohol (PVA) and borate, and this multicellular skin substitutes displayed a linear cellular organization and reduced the formation of a keratinized epidermis that resembles normal skin [133]; Braziulis et al. treated collagen hydrogels by plastic compression and yielded ideal mechanical and biological performances [134]. Jeong et al. proved the influence of stiffness on the dermal fibroblasts cultured in collagen hydrogels crosslinked with poly(ethylene glycol) disuccinmidylester. They found that a cell-encapsulating hydrogel with elastic modulus (E) of 1.6 kPa created dermis-like tissue with large amount of GAG and density of blood vessels, while a construct with E of 0.7 kPa generated scar-like tissue [135].

Collagen-based Hydrogels Applied in Heart and Vascular Tissue Engineering

Most of the engineered tissue requires blood vessel networks capable of forming rapidly in a variety of ECM environments, thus the matrix to form neovascular networks is extensively studied. Allen et al. tested and found that the microvascular networks could be formed in type I collagen, fibril and an engineered peptide hydrogel with human endothelial progenitor cells and mesenchymal progenitor cells embedded [136]. De Moraes et al. improved the mechanical and biological performance of collagen hydrogels for vascular tissue engineering by conjugating fibroin microfibers [137]. Duan et al. fabricated hybrid hydrogel composed of native heart matrix and collagen, and found it can induce cardiac differentiation of human embryonic stem cells *in vitro* without the addition of soluble factors [138]. Chiu et al. fabricated an implantable contractile cardiac tissue based on collagen-chitosan hydrogels with microgrooves. The hydrogels were seeded with cardiomyocytes and stimulated with biphasic square pulses. The results indicated that the cell alignment is important to the cardiac function and a smaller groove width is necessary for cells to communicate [139].

Collagen-based Hydrogels Applied in Corneal Tissue Engineering

May Griffith's group reported fabrication method of corneal substitute by several different crosslinker, including carbodiimides (EDC: N-(3-dimethylaminopropyl)- N'-ethylcarbodiimide, and CMC: N-Cyclohexyl- N'-(2-morpholinoethyl) carbodiimide metho-p-toluenesulfonate), epoxy-based crosslinker (BDDGE: 1,4-butanediol diglycidyl ether) [140-142]. And recently, they reported stable corneal regeneration four years after implantation of a cell-free recombinant human collagen type III scaffold (RHC) [143]. Although the RHC is different form the bovine type I collagen, the successful application of collagen-based hydrogel is an inspiration to corneal tissue engineering. One of the most important properties for corneal substitute is the optical transmittance. Meanwhile, the mechanical strength and stability of the hydrogel is high required. Builles et al. reproduced the highly organized architecture of the corneal stroma by using collagen fibrils, which were orthogonally aligned multilayers and prepared by a high magnetic field. Human hemicorneas (stroma + epithelium) was reconstructed in vitro with the scaffold. The *in vivo* experiments showed this orthogonally oriented multilayer collagen hydrogel could be used to repair the anterior region of the stroma, leading to re-epithelialization and recovery of both transparency and ultrastructural organization [144]. Deng et al. fabricated interpenetrating polymer network (IPN) collagen and 6-methacryloyl-α-D-galactopyranose hydrogels by simultaneously photocuring and chemically crosslinking, with the help of PEG diacrylate and EDC/NHS. The optical characteristics and mechanical properties of the IPN hydrogels, together with the results of in vitro experiments, indicated the promising application in corneal lamellar keratoplasty [145]. Mi and Connon et al. prepared photochemically cross-linked plastically compressed collagen hydrogels to support corneal epithelial cells [146-148]. Li et al. investigated the morphologic characteristics and proliferation of rabbit corneal stromal cells on collagen-chitosan- sodium hyaluronate under simulated microgravity [149]. Giasson et al. constructed stromal equivalents by seeding fibroblasts in a collagen hydrogel on which epithelial and endothelial cells were added on each side, to test the presenting of adherent junction proteins. They drew the conclusion that the collagen-based corneal equivalent simulated the native cornea and the presence of cell-cell contacts because of cells from epithelial and endothelial layers expressed adherent junction proteins [150].

Collagen-based Hydrogels Applied in other Soft Tissue Engineering

The application of collagen-based hydrogels has extended to other soft tissue engineering, including tracheal tissue, lung tissue, hepatic tissue, neural tissue and so on. Naito et al. reported a novel tracheal tissue engineering technology *in vitro* and *in vivo* for the first time. The bioartificial trachea was fabricated from fibroblast and collagen hydrogels, mechanically supported by osteogenically- induced MSC in ring-shaped 3D-hydrogel cultures, and was applied in an experimental model of rat trachea injury [151]. Dunphy et al. improved the mechanical properties of collagen hydrogels by adding elastin to meet the requirement of a single alveolar wall. The composite hydrogels with seeding lung fibroblasts were found to have a stiffness equal to the theoretical value for a single alveolar wall (approximate to 5kPa) [152]. Zhao et al. prepared engineered hepatic units using collagen hydrogel, and achieved 3D vascularized hepatic tissue *in vivo* [153]. Lee et al. prepared collagen hydrogel combined with mesoporous nanoparticles loading nerve growth factor to improve the neurite outgrowth of cells [154]. Martens et al. fabricated collagen hydrogel containing aligned columns of dental pulp stem cells, and further guided the neurite outgrowth [155].

Collagen-based Hydrogels Applied in Cartilage Tissue Engineering

As a strong and elastic connective tissue, cartilage plays an important role in human body. With no blood vessels and low cell density, the cartilage defect with a certain volume can hardly be self-healing. Except a small part of the cartilage is composed of chondrocytes, the main constituents are the hydrated extracellular matrix with collagens and proteoglycans. Although the hyaline cartilage of human body is well understood both in constituents and structure, researchers still believe that remarkable little quantitative information is available with respect to the biochemical constituents in (fibro)cartilaginous tissues, such as collagen content, or the various posttranslational modifications of collagen [156]. Vonk et al. noticed that the tissue engineering strategies to replace cartilaginous tissues pay in general little attention to the biochemical differences of the tissues or the phenotypical differences of the chondrocytes under consideration. They analyzed the quantitative biochemical data of the cartilaginous tissues, and provided data on mRNA levels from chondrocytes. They found the expression levels of genes involved in the cross-linking of collagen were different cells isolated from various cartilaginous tissues. They concluded that more markers could be used for cartilage tissue engineering, but not only type II collagen and aggrecan [156].

Tissue engineering is considered to be an ideal treatment for cartilage defect repair and regeneration [157]. Autologous chondrocyte implantation (ACI) is one of the most successful biomedical treatments in the cartilage tissue engineering. Since the first performed in Sweden in 1987, ACI attracted great attentions and spread to clinical application worldwide. Briefly, the ACI take places in two stages. Firstly, a small amount of cartilage is sampled from the patient and the chondrocytes are isolated by enzyme. Following, the cells are cultured *in vitro* for 4-6 weeks and proliferated to enough population to re-implant on the damaged area of cartilage. After that, the patient undergoes the second treatment, which needs an open-knee surgery. During the implantation, the cells are seeded on a tibial periosteum or collagen membrane and then applied on the damaged area. The details of ACI are developed in decades, including preoperative assessment, surgical techniques (exposure, defect preparation, graft preparation and fixation and so on) and postoperative rehabilitation, and improvements and influencing factors are further studied and summarized [158-161]. With a history of nearly 30 years, long-term outcome of ACI is follow-up and evaluated by quantitative magnetic resonance imaging techniques or other assessments. For examples, Peterson et al., reported full-thickness cartilage lesions of the knee treated by ACI after 10-20 years long-term results [162]; Pelissier et al. evaluated the defect quality of the first-generation ACI technique with 10 years MRI results [163]; and Niemeyer et al. reported 13-17 years long-term outcomes after first-generation ACI to found satisfying clinical results [164]. However, ACI is unsatisfied and further evolved to another treatment of articular cartilage defect repair -- matrix-induced autologous chondrocyte implantation (MACI) was improved based on ACI and advanced in the latest decade. Ebert et al. studied the correlation between clinical and radiological or MRI outcomes 5 years after MACI [165, 166], and predictive factors [167]. Enea et al. investigated the quality of the repaired tissue and the relationship between histological outcome and the macroscopic appearance in the knee [168] and patellofemoral joint [169]. At the same time, Hindle et al. studied the effect of handling the collagen membrane during MACI on the viability of implanted chondrocytes [170]. Schneider et al. tried to improve the MACI by replacing the membrane by collagen hydrogel (CaReS) and confirmed it was a safe and clinically effective treatment [171].

Even with the great progress of ACI and MACI in the cartilage tissue engineering, the drawbacks of these treatments are illustrated, such as the need of open-knee surgery, long term *in vitro* culture of chondrocytes with limited cell passages etc. The booming developments of mesenchymal stem cell (MSC) treatments in the recent decade make it possible to repair the cartilage defect by chondrogensis of MSC based on novel biomaterials. Akgun et al. compared the outcomes of matrix-induced autologous MSC implantation with MACI for the treatment of isolated chondral defects of the knee. And they concluded that the former treatment can be used effectively and may potentially accelerate recovery [172]. Meanwhile, arthroscope was applied to have minimal invasive treatment and compared with open MACI [173].

Except the clinical application of collagen-based biomaterials mentioned above in cartilage tissue engineering, some more materials and techniques are under developing. Some researches try to fabricate the materials based on synthetic polymers. Even providing appropriate tensile strength, synthetic polymer substrates still need to be improved by collagen grafting or coating to improve the cell attachments and phenotypes. For example, Cai et al. fabricated 3D PCL scaffolds by eletrohydrodynamic printing and grafted by collagen with the mediation of polydoamine, and the culture of seeded chondrocytes shown favorable results [174]. Chen et al. prepared PCL scaffold with pre-designed macro and micro features by selective laser sintering, and further hybridized with collagen hydrogel for cartilage tissue engineering [175]. Dai et al. prepared PLGA knitted meshes and formed collagen microsponge in interstices or one side of the mesh or between two meshes [176]. Compared to the synthetic polymers, the natural polymers show a better biocompatibility and biofunctions. Kwon et al. compared the responses of chondrocyte, which were seeded within three polymeric materials including silk, collagen and PLA, to Il-1 β and TNF α. They concluded that the silk and collagen scaffolds might regulate gene expression and response to inflammatory stimuli in chondrocytes [157]. Since the compositions of extracellular matrix in cartilage are mainly collagen and glycosaminoglycan, including hyaluronic acid and chondroitin sulfate, more natural polymer based cartilage tissue engineering medical products are fabricated and further studied the potential in cartilage regeneration. However, the hyaluronic-based and collagen-based cartilage repair materials perform differently both in research and application. Welsch et al. compared cartilage repair tissue at the femoral condyle noninvasively after matrix-associated autologous chondrocyte transplantation using Hyalograft C, a hyaluronic-based scaffold, and CaReS, a collagen-based scaffold, with magnetic resonance imaging using morphologic scoring and T2 mapping. They concluded that both repair tissues provided comparable results in most morphologic parameters. However, collagen scaffold repaired cartilage tissue shown better in the surface and higher T2 values [177].

The combination of collagen hydrogel and chondrocyte is broadly studied to improve the ACI or novel treatments. To find the preference of cartilage repair hydrogels, Rutgers et al. compared the different effect of collagen type I or type II on chondrogensis by cultured human articular chondrocytes. They concluded that the chondrocyte cultured on both collagen type I and type II promoted more active matrix production and no significant differences were observed [178]. Berendsen et al. investigated the effect of collagen type I and type II on the matrix contraction and relative gene expression levels of matrix proteins and MMPs. They found that the collagen composition of the hydrogels affected matrix contraction by articular chondrocytes [179]. Gavenis et al. evaluated the potential value of a cell-free collagen hydrogel plug for the treatment of focal cartilage defects with the help of arthroscope, and they found it led to a good quality repair tissue in the nude mouse model [180]. Mueller-Rath improved the collagen hydrogel biomechanical property by condensation of the gel and evaluated the biochemical properties. Chondrocytes seeded within the condense collagen hydrogel were able to produce ECM and showed proliferation [181]. Puetzer et al. confirmed the high density collagen hydrogel had advantages in both biochemical and mechanical properties when seeded with meniscal fibrochondrocytes and cultured *in vitro* for 4 weeks than alginate hydrogel did [182].

Another way to enhance the mechanical property or improve the performance of the collagen hydrogel is crosslinking or blending with other polymers to form interpenetrating polymeric network (IPN). As reported by Makris et al., hypoxia and lysyl oxidase-induced crosslinking were effective to improve the hydrogel properties. The conclusion holds promise toward applying hypoxia and lysyl oxidase at precise point in time to promote tensile integrity and direct construct maturation [183, 184]. Deponti et al. developed collagen hydrogels seeded with chondrocytes and optimized the seeding process by addition of the fibrin glue. The proper culture time (at least 3 weeks) for ideal scaffold maturation *in vitro* are achieved [185]. Yang et al. demonstrated that a collagen-based solid fibrous capsule would enhance the early integration of engineered and native cartilage tissues [186]. Chicatun et al. prepared dense collagen/ chitosan hydrogels to discover the positive effect of incorporated chitosan [187]. Guo et al. prepared the IPN hydrogels of collagen/chondroitin sulfate/hyaluronic acid via two simultaneous processes of collagen self-assembly and crosslinking polymerization of chondroitin sulfate-methacrylate and hyaluronic acid-methacrylate. The results suggested that the IPN hydrogels upregulated cartilage specific gene expression and promoted the secreting of GAG and collagen II [188].

With the development of equipments or facilities, more devices are employed to the fabrication and application of collagen-based hydrogels for cartilage regeneration. Li et al. studied the effect of insulin-like growth factor-1 and basic fibroblast growth factor on the proliferation of chondrocytes embedded in the collagen hydrogel using an integrated microfluidic device. With the device, the experimental conditions were flexible and a smaller number of cells were required [189]. Rosenzweig et al. compared the primary chondrocytes seeded in dense collagen hydrogels on continuously expanding culture dishes with that on static silicone dishes. The results indicated that the continuously expanding method produced more cartilaginous matrix with superior mechanical properties [190]. Nebelung et al. employed long-term cyclic or continuous compressive loading on collagen hydrogels to modulate the biological and mechanical properties and the responses of chondrocytes embedded [191, 192].

In addition, the researches on collagen hydrogels embedded with mesenchymal stem cell (MSC) and the controlling of differentiation fate of MSC are interesting topics in recent years [193]. MSC were found chondrogenic differentiated in collagen hydrogels both *in vitro* and *in vivo* without growth factors [194, 195], but no chondrogenic differentiation was observed within collagen sponge [196]. The chondrogenic differentiation was further researched from both materials and culture conditions aspects. Meng et al. discovered that the ATDC5 and human MSC could be chondrogenic differentiated when seeded in tricalcium phosphate-collagen-hyaluronan scaffold and cultured in basal medium without any exogenous growth factors *in vitro* [197]. Chen et al. embedded human umbilical cord derived MSC (UC-MSC) within collagen hydrogel and the constructs were induced in standard chondrocyte conditioning medium. The real-time PCR, histochemistry and immunohistochemistry analyses demonstrated that the collagen hydrogel could provide an appropriate 3D environment for the chondrogenesis of UC-MSC [198]. Dinescu et al. prepared collagen-sericin scaffolds improved with hyaluronic acid and chondroitin sulfate, and the hydrogel were seeded with human adipose derived stem cells and the biological performances were positively evaluated [199]. As introduced in the literature, there are many researches focus on the chondrogenic differentiation of MSC, and an effective and economical method is still under research.

Collagen-based Hydrogels Applied in Osteochondral and Bone Tissue Engineering

Even though hydrogels were considered not suitable for the bone regeneration owing to their incapable of surviving and bearing mechanical load *in vivo*, there are still some researches trying to understand the cell biology of osteoprogenitor cells embedded in hydrogels, especially during the cell differentiation and maturation. Damaraju et al. applied mechanical load to impart confined compression to collagen hydrogels seeded with murine embryonic stem cells, and cell responses as they were stimulated at 5-30 days were examined. They found the mechanical stimulation resulted in significant different in the structure and organization of mineralization presented in the collagen hydrogels; and some of the samples produced a highly structured honeycomb-shaped mineralization in the matrix, which was indicative of late osteoblast/early osteocyte activity [200]. While collagen is normally applied as surface modifier on inorganic ceramics or metal substrates for bone tissue engineering, more researches are conducted on the collagen composite scaffolds for osteochondral tissue. Ouyang's group investigated different methods for osteochondral defect healing, including bi-layer collagen/microporous electrospun nanofiber scaffold [201], combination of parathyroid hormone-related protein and collagen-silk scaffold [202], and collagen scaffold with horizontal and vertical oriented channels along with stromal cell-derived factor-1 [203]. Collagen and hydroxyapatite or tricalcium phosphates are another generally combined to fabricate composite scaffold for osteochondral repair. Zhou et al. produced collagen-hydroxyapatite scaffold with different integrated layers and studied the in vitro generation of osteochondral differentiation of MSC [204]. Maehara et al. carried out a similar research with fibroblast growth factor-2 impregnated to repair large osteochondral defects in a rabbit model [205]. Zheng et al. reported a triple-phased composite hydrogel synthesized in situ by collagen, alginate and nano-hydroxyapatite, and demonstrated this composite hydrogels held promise in osteochondral regeneration [206].

4.3. Other Fundamental Research on Collagen and Collagen-Based Biomaterials

Collagen and collagen-based biomaterials are so widely studied that not only the preparation and application are included, but also mechanism and derivatives are covered. The new understandings on bioactive sites/segments of collagen and cell-collagen interactions will be beneficial to the development of fabrication and application of collagen and collagen-based biomaterials. These researches will tamp the fundament for collagen science, and guide the studies of other natural polymers too. Briefly, we will review parts of the fundamental researches conducting at present.

Collagen Structure and Its Relationship with Biological Performance

The characteristics of collagen originate from its particular primary structure and triple helix structure in a great degree. Although the amino acid types and sequence of the collagen is completely analyzed and well understood, the spatial structure of collagen is hard to examine quantitatively and promptly because it is varied at the different stages of biosynthesis and may be transformed during the preparation or application. Owing to the excellent biological performance of collagen is principally depended on the 3D structure of collagen, the researches on collagen structure is always under implementing, especially when it concerns to the neo-tissue formation and regeneration. Understanding the complex structure of collagen should provide new insights into tissue growth, development, regeneration and disease [207]. As early as 2002, Leikina et al. had a suspicion that the collagen in physiological solution is a random coil rather than a triple helix, which is an energetically preferred conformation of collagen and is a widely held belief. They measured the human lung collagen monomers denatured at 37°C within a couple of days, and the unfolding was observed even below 36 °C. Thus, they believed that collagen helices would begin to unfold once secreted from cells. Refolding of full length and native triple helices occurred only below 30 °C. They concluded that type I collagen is thermally unstable at body temperature [208]. Dr. Joseph P. R. O. Orgel focused on the research of collagen structure for a long period. They presented a crystallographic determination (X-ray diffraction) of collagen type I supermolecular structure, where the molecular conformation of each collagen segment found within the naturally occurring crystallographic unit cell had been defined. This structure showed that the molecular packing topology of the collagen molecule was such that packing neighbors were arranged to form a supertwisted (discontinuous) right-handed microfibril that interdigitates with neighboring microfibrils [209]. Although the packing structure underwent debating [210], it still could be used with care due to the intrinsic limitations [211]. With the utilization of x-ray diffraction and atomic force microscopy, they recognized the most crucial functional domains in collagen, which localized primarily to the overlap region ("master control region"). Also, their results indicated there was a constellation of "cryptic" sequence, which was hidden beneath the fibril surface, poised to promote hemostasis and cell-collagen interactions in tissue injury and regeneration [212]. In recent years, they discussed helical symmetry in collagen structure by comparing X-ray diffraction data collected from type I and type II containing tissues, since the symmetry question related to extracellular matrix organization and cellular integration [213]. Chen et al. established a second-harmonic generation (SHG) microscopy to study collagen fibril/fiber structure, and they considered that the SHG was a powerful modality for imaging fibrillar collagen in a diverse range of tissues [214]. Later, Cicchi et al. expressed similar point of views [215]. Mercado et al. investigated the feasibility of using high-frequency quantitative ultrasound to characterize collagen microstructure nondestructively [216]. As one of the most significant feature of type I collagen fibril, people studied D-spacing to understand the structure and function in collagen. Wallace and Fang et al. introduced a quantitative method to measure the D-periodic spacing of type I collagen fibrils using atomic force microscopy and 2D fast Fourier transform approach, and determined the D-spacing of collagen from different cellular origin or anatomical location, namely teeth, dermis, bones and tendons. They found that the mean D-spacing values are not statistically significant but the distribution of D-spacing is significant [217, 218]. Further, Erickson et al. compared the morphology of normal type I collagen with that in disease models, they demonstrated that it is the D-spacing distribution but not the D-spacing mean showed significant differences in estrogen depletion [219]. However, Su et al. found that the D-spacing was homogeneous in a single type I collagen fibril or in different fibril bundles, which had value of 67nm and narrow distribution of 2.5nm but not 10nm as Wallace et al. determined [220]. The further investigation is still under discussion [221, 222].

Computer assisted modeling of collagen microfibril model is an effective method to study the structure of collagen. Along with more understanding of collagen structure, the collagen microfibril models are gradually established. Computer-assistant research is beneficial to understand three-dimensional structure of collagen (micro)fibril and fiber, also it is helpful to find the possible bioactive sites or segments in collagen. The achievements may be crucial to understand the mechanism of cell-collagen interactions and guide design and fabrication of the novel generation of collagen-based tissue engineering medical products. Israelowitz et al. established a model of type I collagen fibrils by using Protein Data Bank and TissueLab software, and further collagen fibers and 3D matrices were created [223]. Brown built a bovine type I collagen microfibril model, which was comprised of five right-handed triple helices in a left-handed super coil containing gap and overlap regions as well as the nonhelical telopeptides. This model was applied to predict or visualize chemistry to stabilize the matrix, insert an active agent or otherwise modify collagen [224]. Soares et al. hypothesized that the cellular contractile stresses were responsible for collagen orientation, and they established a computational model to describe the collagen orientation in statically cultured engineered tissues. The model described the cellular α-actin turnover and the stresses developed by them were integrated in a structural constitutive model describing the mechanical behavior of collagen fibers [225].

New Sources for Collagen Preparation

The potential risks of animal-derived collagen make people cautious to the application of collagen-based biomaterials. To avoid the hazards of TSE and other viruses carried in bovine or pig, researchers searching for new sources for collagen preparation. Collagen derived from alternative and riskless sources is required, and marine organisms are among the safe and recently exploited ones. In the latest years, marine origin collagens have drawn the attentions a lot [226, 227]. Fernandes-Silva et al. prepared collagen from shark skin and further fabricated the scaffold. After crosslinking with genipin under high pressure carbon dioxide, the chondrocyte-like cell line was seeded in the scaffold and cultured *in vitro* [228]. Di Benedetto et al. prepared collagen from the peristomial membrane of thesea urchin *Paracentrotus lividus*, and the in vitro tests shown a good biocompatibility on prepared collagen [229]. Ramanathan et al. extracted collagen from the fish skin of *Arothron stellatus*, and the physical, chemical and biological properties suggested its potential in tissue engineering [230]. Marine derived collagen is extracted from many different kinds of marine fishes, and several of them have been applied in the research of tissue engineering. Lin et al. studied the application potentiality of *Callyspongiidae* marine sponge in bone tissue engineering [231]. Krishnan et al. prepared and evaluated collagen from fish scales, and in vitro cultured with limbal stem cell. The evaluation results were compared with human amniotic membrane [232]. Pallela et al. prepared a scaffold containing chitosan, hydroxyapatite and *Ircina fusca* derived marine sponge collagen, and the scaffold was characterized biophysicochemically in bone regeneration applications [233]. Bermueller et al. evaluated the marine collagen for application in nasal cartilage repair. They prepared the collagen construct and applied in animal model for nasal septum repair to find positive results [234]. Hoyer et al. fabricated collagen scaffold, which was prepared from the jellyfish *Rhopilema esculentum*, and seeded with human mesenchymal stem cells to investigate the biological performance. The results illustrated that the SOX9, collagen type II and aggrecan were upregulated after *in vitro* chondrogenic stimulated culture [235].

Another incredible novel resource for collagen preparation is transgenic plants, which is reported by scientists from France and Israel. Ruggiero et al. reported that constructs were engineered from cDNA encoding the human proα1(I) chain to generate transgenic tobacco plants expressing collagen I, and Large amounts of recombinant collagen were purified from field grown plant material [236]. In recent years, Shoseyov et al. introduced that the plant extracted recombinant human collagen type I forms thermally stable helical structures, fibrillates, and demonstrates bioactivity resembling that of native collagen [237, 238]. With the plant-derived human collagen, they fabricated electrospun nonwoven scaffolds and lyophilized sponges, and studied the potential for skin tissue engineering [239].

Collagen Derived Polypeptide and Collagen Mimetic Peptide

During the process of elucidating the collagen triple helix and the factors responsible for its stabilization, collagen derived polypeptide or collagen mimetic peptide (CMP) was initially developed and studied. Following, the biologists and polymer chemists produced CMP based nanostructured fibrous scaffolds as the building blocks of tissue engineering. Although, there is a burst of research on recreating higher order assembly and biological function of native collagen based on CMP, most of the research is still at an early stage [240, 241]. With the development of modern synthesis methods and particular ligation chemistries basing on activated ester, carbodiimide chemistry etc., versatile CMP and CMP-collagen or CMP-polymer conjugates are prepared and investigated [242]. Yu's group synthesized CMP [$(ProHypGly)_7$-Tyr] and introduced photoactive function groups. This photopolymerizable CMP derivative was copolymerized with poly(ethylene oxide) diacrylate to create covalent crosslinking hydrogels, showing outstanding histology and immunohistochemistry performance after seeded with chondrocytes and *in vitro* cultured for 2 weeks [243]. Then, Li et al. prepared a single-stranded CMP (sequence: $(GlyProHyp)_9$) which can conjugate to common fluorophores (carboxyfluorescein). Then, the CMP conjugation can bind to collagen chain by triple helix hybridization. By staining with labeled CMP, both intact and MMP-1 cleaved collagen chain could be detected even more effectively than anticollagen I antibody [244]. They further applied this CMP to stabilize conducting polymer nanoparticles for collagen targeting [245]. Seeking for an ideal design method of biomimetic collagen for tissue engineering, Krishnamoorthy et al. described a bottom-up approach to design two computationally mutated molecular models that used non-covalent interactions to crosslink triple helices of tropocollagen molecules and thus promote self-association [246]. Sarkar et al. reported a strategy, which depended on the formation of a staggered triple helical species facilitated by interchain charged pairs, to design peptides can self-assembly into fibers. They synthesized F0 [$(PKG)_4(POG)_4(DOG)_4$], F1 [$(PKG)_4(DOG)_4(POG)_4$] and F2 [$(PKG)_4(PKG)_4(DOG)_4$] and found that F0, F1 and F2 all self-assembled into collagen-like nanofibers, but F0 formed a clear hydrogel with good viscoelastic properties while fibers from F1 and F2 phase separated and precipitated. Accordingly, they demonstrated that the nature of the sticky-ended intermediate had dramatic effect on the supramolecular assembly and solubility of CMP [247].

Summary and Perspectives

As one of the most abundant molecules in vertebrates, type I collagen constituting major parts of the fibrillar extracellular matrix, thus providing structural integrity and mechanical resilience. It has therefore become an almost ubiquitous biomolecule to use in contemporary biomimetic cell culture scaffolds and in tissue engineering scenarios, where new functions for biomedical applications are sought. Bovine type I collagen has various advantages and will be widely applied as the main material for tissue engineering in a relatively long period. The preparation, characterization and application of collagen and collagen-based biomaterials in this chapter represent selected examples in the extensive advancing researches. Without any doubt, the robust techniques and approaches to use collagen with or without modification, and the schemes to mimic the key features of the natural extracellular matrix will be the further goals and challenges for studies of collagen and collagen-based biomaterials. By making a breakthrough of native collagen academically or practically, essential progress will be made for collagen-based biomaterials or devices. More collagen-based medical products for tissue regeneration will be evaluated in the clinical trials with effectively control of the risks, and even more novel products and techniques will move their way through preclinical investigation toward clinical application. These creative products will enable new biosurgical approaches in tissue regeneration, and will expand the regenerative methods for repairing and replacing defective or damaged tissues.

References

[1] Chen, G., et al., Effect of internal structure of collagen/hydroxyapatite scaffold on the osteogenic differentiation of mesenchymal stem cells. *Curr Stem Cell Res Ther,* 2015. *10*(2): p. 99-108.

[2] Gelse, K., E. Poschl, and T. Aigner, Collagens--structure, function, and biosynthesis. *Adv Drug Deliv Rev,* 2003. *55*(12): p. 1531-46.

[3] Koide, T. and K. Nagata, Collagen biosynthesis. *Collagen,* 2005. *247*: p. 85-114.

[4] Canty, E.G. and K.E. Kadler, Collagen fibril biosynthesis in tendon: a review and recent insights. *Comparative Biochemistry and Physiology a-Molecular and Integrative Physiology, 2002. 133*(4): p. 979-985.

[5] Shoulders, M.D. and R.T. Raines, Collagen structure and stability. *Annu Rev Biochem,* 2009. *78*: p. 929-58.

[6] UniProt, *CO1A1_BOVIN*, UniProt. http://www.uniprot.org/uniprot/P02453

[7] ASTM F2212-11, Standard Guide for Characterization of Type I Collagen as Starting Material for Surgical Implants and Substrates for Tissue Engineered Medical Products (TEMPs), ASTM International, West Conshohocken, PA.

[8] McClain, P.E. and E.R. Wiley, Differential scanning calorimeter studies of the thermal transitions of collagen. Implications on structure and stability. *J Biol Chem,* 1972. *247*(3): p. 692-7.

[9] Bozec, L. and M. Odlyha, Thermal Denaturation Studies of Collagen by Microthermal Analysis and Atomic Force Microscopy. *Biophysical Journal,* 2011. *101*(1): p. 228-236.

[10] Fallas, J.A., L.E.R. O'Leary, and J.D. Hartgerink, Synthetic collagen mimics: self-assembly of homotrimers, heterotrimers and higher order structures. *Chemical Society Reviews,* 2010. *39*(9): p. 3510-3527.

[11] Khew, S.T. and Y.W. Tong, The Specific Recognition of a Cell Binding Sequence Derived from Type I Collagen by Hep3B and L929 Cells. *Biomacromolecules,* 2007. *8*(10): p. 3153-3161.

[12] Quan, B.D. and E.D. Sone, Cryo-TEM analysis of collagen fibrillar *structure. Methods Enzymol,* 2013. *532*: p. 189-205.

[13] ISO, *ISO 10993 Biological evaluation of medical devices Part 1: Evaluation and testing within a risk management process.* 2009, International Organization for Standardization: Switzerland.

[14] ISO, *ISO 10993 Biological evaluation of medical devices Part 5: Tests for in vitro cytotoxicity.* 2009, International Organization for Standardization: Switzerland.

[15] ISO, *ISO 10993 Biological evaluation of medical devices Part 10: Tests for irritation and skin sensitization.* 2010, International Organization for Standardization: Switzerland.

[16] ISO, *ISO 10993 Biological evaluation of medical devices Part 11: Tests for systemic toxicity.* 2006, International Organization for Standardization: Switzerland.

[17] ISO, *ISO 10993 Biological evaluation of medical devices Part 3: Tests for genotoxicity, carcinogenicity and reproductive toxicity.* 2014, International Organization for Standardization: Switzerland.

[18] ISO, *ISO 10993 Biological evaluation of medical devices Part 6: Tests for local effects after implantation.* 2007, International Organization for Standardization: Switzerland.

[19] ISO, *ISO 10993 Biological evaluation of medical devices Part 9: Framework for identification and quantification of potential degradation products.* 2009, International Organization for Standardization: Switzerland.

[20] ISO, *ISO 10993 Biological evaluation of medical devices Part 13: Identification and quantification of degradation products from polymeric medical devices.* 2010, International Organization for Standardization: Switzerland.

[21] Bae, J.e., et al., Virus Inactivation during the Manufacture of a Collagen Type I from Bovine Hides. *Korean Journal of Microbiology*, 2012. *48*(4): p. 314-318.

[22] Ferreira, A.M., et al., Collagen for bone tissue regeneration. *Acta Biomaterialia,* 2012. *8*(9): p. 3191-3200.

[23] Sarker, B., et al., Collagen/silica nanocomposites and hybrids for bone tissue engineering. *Nanotechnology Reviews,* 2013. *2*(4): p. 427-447.

[24] Mafi, P., et al., Evaluation of Biological Protein-Based Collagen Scaffolds in Cartilage and Musculoskeletal Tissue Engineering- A Systematic Review of the Literature. *Current Stem Cell Research & Therapy,* 2012. *7*(4): p. 302-309.

[25] Zhao, J. and M. Li, *Application of collagen composite scaffold in vascular tissue engineering.* Zhongguo xiu fu chong jian wai ke za zhi = Zhongguo xiufu chongjian waike zazhi = Chinese journal of reparative and reconstructive surgery, 2011. *25*(7): p. 859-62.

[26] Gaspar, A., et al., Collagen-based scaffolds for skin tissue engineering. *Journal of medicine and life,* 2011. *4*(2): p. 172-7.

[27] McMillan, J.R., Comparison of polymer and collagen based skin tissue engineering scaffolds. *Experimental Dermatology,* 2011. *20*(10): p. E874-E874.

[28] Chattopadhyay, S. and R.T. Raines, Collagen-Based Biomaterials for Wound Healing. *Biopolymers,* 2014. *101*(8): p. 821-833.

[29] Parenteau-Bareil, R., R. Gauvin, and F. Berthod, Collagen-Based Biomaterials for Tissue Engineering Applications. *Materials,* 2010. *3*(3): p. 1863-1887.

[30] Brown, R.A., In the beginning there were soft collagen-cell gels: towards better 3D connective tissue models? *Experimental Cell Research,* 2013. *319*(16): p. 2460-2469.

[31] Liu, Y., et al., One-Step Derivation of Mesenchymal Stem Cell (MSC)-Like Cells from Human Pluripotent Stem Cells on a Fibrillar Collagen Coating. *Plos One,* 2012. *7*(3).

[32] Tu, J., et al., Preparation and antibiotic drug release of mineralized collagen coatings on titanium. *J Mater Sci Mater Med,* 2012. *23*(10): p. 2413-23.

[33] Lafisco, M., et al., Electrospun Collagen Mimicking the Reconstituted Extracellular Matrix Improves Osteoblastic Differentiation Onto Titanium Surfaces. *Journal of Nanoscience and Nanotechnology,* 2013. *13*(7): p. 4720-4726.

[34] Wang, Q.Q., et al., Preparation of a HA/collagen film on a bioactive titanium surface by the electrochemical deposition method. *Biomed Mater,* 2011. *6*(5): p. 055009.

[35] Li, Y., et al., Collagen coated tantalum substrate for cell proliferation. *Colloids and Surfaces B-Biointerfaces,* 2012. *95*: p. 10-15.

[36] Zhao, N. and D.H. Zhu, Collagen Self-Assembly on Orthopedic Magnesium Biomaterials Surface and Subsequent Bone Cell Attachment. *Plos One,* 2014. *9*(10): p. e110420.

[37] Ebrahimi, S., K. Ghafoori-Tabrizi, and H. Rafii-Tabar, Molecular dynamics simulation of the adhesive behavior of collagen on smooth and randomly rough TiO2 and Al2O3 surfaces. *Computational Materials Science,* 2013. *71*: p. 172-178.

[38] Cai, K., et al., Regulation of endothelial cells migration on poly(D, L-lactic acid) films immobilized with collagen gradients. *Colloids and Surfaces B-Biointerfaces,* 2010. *79*(1): p. 291-297.

[39] Kiran, S., K.C. Nune, and R.D. Misra, The significance of grafting collagen on polycaprolactone composite scaffolds: Processing-structure-functional property relationship. *J Biomed Mater Res* A, 2015.

[40] Sugiyama, K., et al., Coating of collagen on a poly(l-lactic acid) sponge surface for tissue engineering. *Materials Science & Engineering C-Materials for Biological Applications,* 2012. *32*(2): p. 290-295.

[41] Yu, Z., et al., Improvement of intertrochanteric bone quality in osteoporotic female rats after injection of polylactic acid-polyglycolic acid copolymer/collagen type I microspheres combined with bone mesenchymal stem cells. *International Orthopaedics,* 2012. *36*(10): p. 2163-2171.

[42] Kawase, T., et al., Collagen-Coated Poly(L-lactide-co-epsilon-caprolactone) Film: A Promising Scaffold for Cultured Periosteal Sheets. *Journal of Periodontology,* 2010. *81*(11): p. 1653-1662.

[43] Lee, H. and G. Kim, Three-dimensional plotted PCL/beta-TCP scaffolds coated with a collagen layer: preparation, physical properties and in vitro evaluation for bone tissue regeneration. *Journal of Materials Chemistry,* 2011. *21*(17): p. 6305-6312.

[44] Chen, J.-P., S.-F. Li, and Y.-P. Chiang, Bioactive Collagen-Grafted Poly-L-Lactic Acid Nanofibrous Membrane for Cartilage Tissue Engineering. *Journal of Nanoscience and Nanotechnology,* 2010. *10*(8): p. 5393-5398.

[45] Hong, S.G. and G.H. Kim, Mechanically improved electrospun PCL biocomposites reinforced with a collagen coating process: preparation, physical properties, and cellular activity. *Bioprocess Biosyst Eng,* 2013. *36*(2): p. 205-14.

[46] Goncalves, F., M.C. Burrows, and L.H. Catalani, Improvement of collagen immobilization on electrospun PLLA and PCL for better cell attachment and proliferation. *Journal of Tissue Engineering and Regenerative Medicine,* 2012. *6*: p. 163-163.

[47] Lao, L., et al., Mineralization of Collagen-Coated Electrospun Poly(lactide-co-glycolide) Nanofibrous Mesh to Enhance Growth and Differentiation of Osteoblasts and Bone Marrow Mesenchymal Stem Cells. *Advanced Engineering Materials,* 2012. *14*(4): p. B123-B137.

[48] McNeil, S.E., H.R. Griffiths, and Y. Perrie, Polycaprolactone Fibres as a Potential Delivery System for Collagen to Support Bone Regeneration. *Current Drug Delivery,* 2011. *8*(4): p. 448-455.

[49] Gautam, S., et al., Surface modification of nanofibrous polycaprolactone/gelatin composite scaffold by collagen type I grafting for skin tissue engineering. *Materials Science & Engineering C-Materials for Biological Applications,* 2014. *34*: p. 402-409.

[50] Liu, H., et al., Biological response of osteoblast-like UMR-106 cells to the modified PHBV matrix-Effects of porosity and collagen dip coating. *Journal of Biomedical Materials Research Part A,* 2010. *92A*(3): p. 922-930.

[51] Ai, J., et al., Fabrication of Coated-Collagen Electrospun PHBV Nanofiber Film by Plasma Method and Its Cellular Study. *Journal of Nanomaterials,* 2011.

[52] He, X.Y., et al., New method for coupling collagen on biodegradable polyurethane for biomedical application. *Journal of Applied Polymer Science,* 2012. *126*: p. E353-E360.

[53] Miyoshi, H., et al., Cryopreservation of Fibroblasts Immobilized Within a Porous Scaffold: Effects of Preculture and Collagen Coating of Scaffold on Performance of Three-Dimensional Cryopreservation. *Artificial Organs,* 2010. *34*(7): p. 609-614.

[54] Kim, T.G., et al., Microstructured scaffold coated with hydroxyapatite/collagen nanocomposite multilayer for enhanced osteogenic induction of human mesenchymal stem cells. *Journal of Materials Chemistry,* 2010. *20*(40): p. 8927-8933.

[55] Thickett, S.C., et al., Micropatterned substrates made by polymer bilayer dewetting and collagen nanoscale assembly support endothelial cell adhesion. *Soft Matter*, 2012. *8*(39): p. 9996-10007.

[56] Stylianou, A., D. Yova, and E. Alexandratou, Nanotopography of collagen thin films in correlation with fibroblast response. *Journal of Nanophotonics,* 2013. *7*.

[57] Stylianou, A. and D. Yova, Surface nanoscale imaging of collagen thin films by Atomic Force Microscopy. *Materials Science & Engineering C-Materials for Biological Applications,* 2013. *33*(5): p. 2947-2957.

[58] Pastorino, L., et al., Oriented collagen nanocoatings for tissue engineering. *Colloids and Surfaces B-Biointerfaces,* 2014. *114*: p. 372-378.

[59] Bosco, R., et al., Configurational effects of collagen/ALP coatings on enzyme immobilization and surface mineralization. *Applied Surface Science,* 2014. *311*: p. 292-299.

[60] Cooper, T.P. and M.V. Sefton, Fibronectin coating of collagen modules increases in vivo HUVEC survival and vessel formation in SCID mice. *Acta Biomaterialia,* 2011. *7*(3): p. 1072-1083.

[61] Hirata, E., et al., Multiwalled carbon nanotube-coating of 3D collagen scaffolds for bone tissue engineering. *Carbon,* 2011. *49*(10): p. 3284-3291.

[62] Baktur, R., S.-H. Yoon, and S. Kwon, Effects of Multiwalled Carbon Nanotube Reinforced Collagen Scaffolds on the Osteogenic Differentiation of Mesenchymal Stem Cells. *Journal of Nanomaterials,* 2013.

[63] Kim, T., et al., Effect of CNT on collagen fiber structure, stiffness assembly kinetics and stem cell differentiation. *Mater Sci Eng C Mater Biol Appl,* 2015. *49*: p. 281-9.

[64] Kanayama, I., et al., Comparative study of bioactivity of collagen scaffolds coated with graphene oxide and reduced graphene oxide. *International Journal of Nanomedicine,* 2014. *9*: p. 3363-3373.
[65] Yang, H.S., et al., Apatite-Coated Collagen Scaffold for Bone Morphogenetic Protein-2 Delivery. *Tissue Engineering Part A,* 2011. *17*(17-18): p. 2153-2164.
[66] Yang, H.S., et al., Efficient Bone Regeneration Induced by Bone Morphogenetic Protein-2 Released from Apatite-Coated Collagen Scaffolds. *Journal of Biomaterials Science, Polymer Edition,* 2012. *23*(13): p. 1659-71.
[67] Tsai, S.W., et al., Preparation and evaluation of a hyaluronate-collagen film for preventing post-surgical adhesion. *J Int Med Res,* 2005. *33*(1): p. 68-76.
[68] Liu, Y., et al., Collagen films with suitable physical properties and biocompatibility for corneal tissue engineering prepared by ion leaching technique. *Materials Letters,* 2012. *87*: p. 1-4.
[69] Boekema, B.K.H.L., et al., Effect of pore size and cross-linking of a novel collagen-elastin dermal substitute on wound healing. *Journal of Materials Science-Materials in Medicine,* 2014. *25*(2): p. 423-433.
[70] Berahim, Z., et al., Biologic Interaction of Three-Dimensional Periodontal Fibroblast Spheroids With Collagen-Based and Synthetic Membranes. *Journal of Periodontology,* 2011. *82*(5): p. 790-797.
[71] Nocini, P.F., et al., Bi-layered collagen nano-structured membrane prototype (collagen matrix 10826 (R)) for oral soft tissue regeneration: an "in vitro" study. *Clinical Oral Implants Research,* 2013. *24*(6): p. 612-617.
[72] Koseoglu, S., et al., Efficacy of Collagen Membrane Seeded With Autologous Gingival Fibroblasts in Gingival Recession Treatment: A Randomized, Controlled Pilot Study. *Journal of Periodontology,* 2013. *84*(10): p. 1416-1424.
[73] Lammers, G., et al., Construction of a Microstructured Collagen Membrane Mimicking the Papillary Dermis Architecture and Guiding Keratinocyte Morphology and Gene Expression. *Macromolecular Bioscience,* 2012. *12*(5): p. 675-691.
[74] Taraballi, F., et al., Amino and carboxyl plasma functionalization of collagen films for tissue engineering applications. *Journal of Colloid and Interface Science,* 2013. *394*: p. 590-597.

[75] Liu, Y., et al., Preparation and characterization of a novel tobramycin-containing antibacterial collagen film for corneal tissue engineering. *Acta Biomaterialia,* 2014. *10*(1): p. 289-299.
[76] Calderon-Colon, X., et al., Structure and properties of collagen vitrigel membranes for ocular repair and regeneration applications. *Biomaterials,* 2012. *33*(33): p. 8286-95.
[77] Forti, F.L., et al., 1,4-Dioxane enhances properties and biocompatibility of polyanionic collagen for tissue engineering applications. *Journal of Materials Science-Materials in Medicine,* 2011. *22*(8): p. 1901-1912.
[78] Gao, J., et al., A Myocardial Patch Made of Collagen Membranes Loaded with Collagen-Binding Human Vascular Endothelial Growth Factor Accelerates Healing of the Injured Rabbit Heart. *Tissue Engineering Part A,* 2011. *17*(21-22): p. 2739-2747.
[79] Yamano, S., et al., The effect of a bioactive collagen membrane releasing PDGF or GDF-5 on bone regeneration. *Biomaterials,* 2014. *35*(8): p. 2446-2453.
[80] Ho, S.T.B., et al., An electrospun polycaprolactone-collagen membrane for the resurfacing of cartilage defects. *Polymer International,* 2010. *59*(6): p. 808-817.
[81] He, X., et al., Electrospun Collagen/Poly(L-lactic acid-co-epsilon-caprolactone) Hybrid Nanofibrous Membranes Combining with Sandwich Construction Model for Cartilage Tissue Engineering. *Journal of Nanoscience and Nanotechnology,* 2013. *13*(6): p. 3818-3825.
[82] He, X., et al., Electrospun collagen-poly(l-lactic acid-co-epsilon-caprolactone) membranes for cartilage tissue engineering. *Regenerative Medicine,* 2013. *8*(4): p. 425-436.
[83] Liu, S.-J., et al., Electrospun PLGA/collagen nanofibrous membrane as early-stage wound dressing. *Journal of Membrane Science,* 2010. *355*(1-2): p. 53-59.
[84] Steele, T.W.J., et al., Collagen-cellulose composite thin films that mimic soft-tissue and allow stem-cell orientation. *Journal of Materials Science-Materials in Medicine, 2013. 24*(8): p. 2013-2027.
[85] Verissimo, D.M., et al., Polyanionic collagen membranes for guided tissue regeneration: Effect of progressive glutaraldehyde cross-linking on biocompatibility and degradation. *Acta Biomaterialia,* 2010. *6*(10): p. 4011-4018.
[86] Grover, C.N., et al., Crosslinking and composition influence the surface properties, mechanical stiffness and cell reactivity of collagen-based films. *Acta Biomaterialia,* 2012. *8*(8): p. 3080-3090.

[87] Liu, Y., L. Ren, and Y. Wang, Crosslinked collagen-gelatin-hyaluronic acid biomimetic film for cornea tissue engineering applications. *Materials Science & Engineering C-Materials for Biological Applications,* 2013. *33*(1): p. 196-201.
[88] Li, W., et al., Fabrication and characterization of chitosan-collagen crosslinked membranes for corneal tissue engineering. *Journal of Biomaterials Science-Polymer Edition,* 2014. *25*(17): p. 1962-1972.
[89] Wang, K., et al., Preparation and Characterization of Collagen-Chitosan-Chondroitin Sulfate Composite Membranes. *Journal of Membrane Biology,* 2012. *245*(11): p. 707-716.
[90] Sandri, M., et al., A collagen membrane-based engineered heart tissue improves cardiac function in ischemic rat hearts. *Bioinspired Biomimetic and Nanobiomaterials,* 2013. *2*(1): p. 20-27.
[91] Yamauchi, K., et al., Films of collagen crosslinked by S-S bonds: preparation and characterization. *Biomaterials,* 2001. *22*(8): p. 855-63.
[92] Stamov, D.R. and T. Pompe, Structure and function of ECM-inspired composite collagen type I scaffolds. *Soft Matter,* 2012. *8*(40): p. 10200-10212.
[93] Tedder, M.E., et al., Assembly and Testing of Stem Cell-Seeded Layered Collagen Constructs for Heart Valve Tissue Engineering. *Tissue Engineering Part* A, 2011. *17*(1-2): p. 25-36.
[94] Lu, H., et al., Cartilage tissue engineering using funnel-like collagen sponges prepared with embossing ice particulate templates. *Biomaterials,* 2010. *31*(22): p. 5825-5835.
[95] Zhang, Q., et al., Preparation of collagen porous scaffolds with a gradient pore size structure using ice particulates. *Materials Letters,* 2013. *107*: p. 280-283.
[96] Zhang, Q., et al., Pore size effect of collagen scaffolds on cartilage regeneration. *Acta Biomaterialia,* 2014. *10*(5): p. 2005-2013.
[97] Khayyatan, F., et al., Behaviour of Human Induced Pluripotent Stem Cell-Derived Neural Progenitors on Collagen Scaffolds Varied in Freezing Temperature and Laminin Concentration. *Cell Journal,* 2014. *16*(1): p. 53-62.
[98] Amruthwar, S.S., A.D. Puckett, and A.V. Janorkar, Preparation and characterization of novel elastin-like polypeptide-collagen composites. *J Biomed Mater Res* A, 2013. *101*(8): p. 2383-91.
[99] Monjo, M., et al., In vivo performance of absorbable collagen sponges with rosuvastatin in critical-size cortical bone defects. *Acta Biomaterialia,* 2010. *6*(4): p. 1405-1412.

[100] Chow, J.P., et al., Mitigation of diabetes-related complications in implanted collagen and elastin scaffolds using matrix-binding polyphenol. *Biomaterials,* 2013. *34*(3): p. 685-695.
[101] Carlisle, C.R., C. Coulais, and M. Guthold, The mechanical stress-strain properties of single electrospun collagen type I nanofibers. *Acta Biomaterialia,* 2010. *6*(8): p. 2997-3003.
[102] Burck, J., et al., Resemblance of electrospun collagen nanofibers to their native structure. *Langmuir,* 2013. *29*(5): p. 1562-72.
[103] Caves, J.M., et al., Fibrillogenesis in Continuously Spun Synthetic Collagen Fiber. *Journal of Biomedical Materials Research Part B-Applied Biomaterials, 2010. 93B*(1): p. 24-38.
[104] Siriwardane, M.L., et al., Controlled formation of cross-linked collagen fibers for neural tissue engineering applications. *Biofabrication,* 2014. *6*(1).
[105] Hempel, U., et al., Artificial extracellular matrices composed of collagen I and sulfated hyaluronan with adsorbed transforming growth factor beta 1 promote collagen synthesis of human mesenchymal stromal cells. *Acta Biomaterialia,* 2012. *8*(2): p. 659-666.
[106] Lloyd, C., J. Besse, and S. Boyce, Controlled-rate freezing to regulate the structure of collagen-glycosaminoglycan scaffolds in engineered skin substitutes. *J Biomed Mater Res B Appl Biomater,* 2014.
[107] Shen, X., et al., A novel method for the fabrication of homogeneous hydroxyapatite/collagen nanocomposite and nanocomposite scaffold with hierarchical porosity. *Journal of Materials Science-Materials in Medicine,* 2011. *22*(2): p. 299-305.
[108] Xia, Z., M.M. Villa, and M. Wei, A Biomimetic Collagen-Apatite Scaffold with a Multi-Level Lamellar Structure for Bone Tissue Engineering. *J Mater Chem B Mater Biol Med,* 2014. *2*(14): p. 1998-2007.
[109] Xiong, L. and Z. He, Fabrication and Properties of Porous Collagen/Hyaluronic Composite Scaffolds Containing Nano-Bioactive Glass for Tissue Engineering. *Journal of Macromolecular Science Part a-Pure and Applied Chemistry,* 2014. *51*(11): p. 891-897.
[110] Hong, S.-J., et al., Novel Scaffolds of Collagen with Bioactive Nanofiller for the Osteogenic Stimulation of Bone Marrow Stromal Cells. *Journal of Biomaterials Applications,* 2010. *24*(8): p. 733-750.
[111] Zugravu, M.V., et al., Physical properties and in vitro evaluation of collagen-chitosan-calcium phosphate microparticle-based scaffolds for

bone tissue regeneration. *Journal of Biomaterials Applications,* 2013. *28*(4): p. 566-579.

[112] Maghdouri-White, Y., et al., Mammary epithelial cell adhesion, viability, and infiltration on blended or coated silk fibroin-collagen type I electrospun scaffolds. *Materials Science & Engineering C-Materials for Biological Applications,* 2014. *43*: p. 37-44.

[113] Prabhakaran, M.P., E. Vatankhah, and S. Ramakrishna, Electrospun Aligned PHBV/Collagen Nanofibers as Substrates for Nerve Tissue Engineering. *Biotechnology and Bioengineering,* 2013. *110*(10): p. 2775-2784.

[114] Wang, G., et al., Electrospun PLGA-silk fibroin-collagen nanofibrous scaffolds for nerve tissue engineering. *In Vitro Cellular & Developmental Biology-Animal,* 2011. *47*(3): p. 234-240.

[115] Ouyang, Y., et al., Fabrication of Seamless Electrospun Collagen/PLGA Conduits Whose Walls Comprise Highly Longitudinal Aligned Nanofibers for Nerve Regeneration. *Journal of Biomedical Nanotechnology,* 2013. *9*(6): p. 931-943.

[116] Lee, B.-K., et al., End-to-side neurorrhaphy using an electrospun PCL/collagen nerve conduit for complex peripheral motor nerve regeneration. *Biomaterials,* 2012. *33*(35): p. 9027-9036.

[117] Kijenska, E., et al., Electrospun bio-composite P(LLA-CL)/collagen I/collagen III scaffolds for nerve tissue engineering. *Journal of Biomedical Materials Research Part B-Applied Biomaterials,* 2012. *100B*(4): p. 1093-1102.

[118] Timnak, A., et al., Fabrication of nano-structured electrospun collagen scaffold intended for nerve tissue engineering. J*ournal of Materials Science-Materials in Medicine, 2011. 22*(6): p. 1555-1567.

[119] Yu, K., T. Inamoto, and Y. Tabata, Adipose Tissue Formation in Collagen Scaffolds with Different Biodegradabilities. *Journal of Biomaterials Science,* Polymer Edition, 2010. *21*(4): p. 463-76.

[120] Yu, K., et al., In situ adipogenesis in fat tissue augmented by collagen scaffold with gelatin microspheres containing basic fibroblast growth factor. *Journal of Tissue Engineering and Regenerative Medicine,* 2010. *4*(1): p. 55-61.

[121] Caliari, S.R., M.A. Ramirez, and B.A.C. Harley, The development of collagen-GAG scaffold-membrane composites for tendon tissue engineering. *Biomaterials*, 2011. *32*(34): p. 8990-8998.

[122] Tuzlakoglu, K., et al., Design of Nano- and Microfiber Combined Scaffolds by Electrospinning of Collagen onto Starch-Based Fiber

Meshes: A Man-Made Equivalent of Natural Extracellular Matrix. *Tissue Engineering Part* A, 2011. *17*(3-4): p. 463-473.

[123] Bian, W., et al., Fabrication of a bio-inspired beta-Tricalcium phosphate/collagen scaffold based on ceramic stereolithography and gel casting for osteochondral tissue engineering. *Rapid Prototyping Journal,* 2012. *18*(1): p. 68-80.

[124] Antoine, E.E., P.P. Vlachos, and M.N. Rylander, Review of Collagen I Hydrogels for Bioengineered Tissue Microenvironments: Characterization of Mechanics, Structure, and Transport. *Tissue Engineering Part B-Reviews,* 2014. *20*(6): p. 683-696.

[125] Marelli, B., et al., Fabrication of injectable, cellular, anisotropic collagen tissue equivalents with modular fibrillar densities. *Biomaterials,* 2015. *37*: p. 183-193.

[126] Abreu, E.L., M.P. Palmer, and M.M. Murray, Collagen density significantly affects the functional properties of an engineered provisional scaffold. *Journal of Biomedical Materials Research Part A,* 2010. *93A*(1): p. 150-157.

[127] Knight, D.P., et al., In vitro formation by reverse dialysis of collagen gels containing highly oriented arrays of fibrils. *J Biomed Mater Res,* 1998. *41*(2): p. 185-91.

[128] Bessea, L., et al., Production of ordered collagen matrices for three-dimensional cell culture. *Biomaterials,* 2002. *23*(1): p. 27-36.

[129] Brown, R.A., et al., Ultrarapid engineering of biomimetic materials and tissues: Fabrication of nano- and microstructures by plastic compression. *Advanced Functional Materials,* 2005. *15*(11): p. 1762-1770.

[130] Mosser, G., et al., Dense tissue-like collagen matrices formed in cell-free conditions. *Matrix Biology,* 2006. *25*(1): p. 3-13.

[131] Wong, V.W., et al., Engineered Pullulan-Collagen Composite Dermal Hydrogels Improve Early Cutaneous Wound Healing. *Tissue Engineering Part A,* 2011. *17*(5-6): p. 631-644.

[132] Desimone, M.F., et al., In vitro Studies and Preliminary In vivo Evaluation of Silicified Concentrated Collagen Hydrogels. *Acs Applied Materials & Interfaces,* 2011. *3*(10): p. 3831-3838.

[133] Hartwell, R., et al., A novel hydrogel-collagen composite improves functionality of an injectable extracellular matrix. *Acta Biomaterialia,* 2011. *7*(8): p. 3060-3069.

[134] Braziulis, E., et al., Modified Plastic Compression of Collagen Hydrogels Provides an Ideal Matrix for Clinically Applicable Skin

Substitutes. *Tissue Engineering Part C-Methods,* 2012. *18*(6): p. 464-474.

[135] Jeong, J.H., et al., Stiffness-Modulated Water Retention and Neovascularization of Dermal Fibroblast-Encapsulating Collagen Gel. *Tissue Engineering Part A,* 2013. *19*(11-12): p. 1275-1284.

[136] Allen, P., J. Melero-Martin, and J. Bischoff, Type I collagen, fibrin and PuraMatrix matrices provide permissive environments for human endothelial and mesenchymal progenitor cells to form neovascular networks. *Journal of Tissue Engineering and Regenerative Medicine,* 2011. *5*(4): p. E74-E86.

[137] de Moraes, M.A., et al., Mechanical and Biological Performances of New Scaffolds Made of Collagen Hydrogels and Fibroin Microfibers for Vascular Tissue Engineering. *Macromolecular Bioscience,* 2012. *12*(9): p. 1253-1264.

[138] Duan, Y., et al., Hybrid Gel Composed of Native Heart Matrix and Collagen Induces Cardiac Differentiation of Human Embryonic Stem Cells without Supplemental Growth Factors. *Journal of Cardiovascular Translational Research,* 2011. *4*(5): p. 605-615.

[139] Chiu, L.L.Y., K. Janic, and M. Radisic, Engineering of oriented myocardium on three-dimensional micropatterned collagen-chitosan hydrogel. *International Journal of Artificial Organs,* 2012. *35*(4): p. 237-250.

[140] Islam, M.M., M. Griffith, and K. Merrett, Fabrication of a human recombinant collagen-based corneal substitute using carbodiimide chemistry. *Methods in molecular biology (Clifton, N.J.),* 2013. *1014*: p. 157-64.

[141] Jae-Il, A., et al., Crosslinked collagen hydrogels as corneal implants: Effects of sterically bulky vs. non-bulky carbodiimides as crosslinkers. *Acta Biomaterialia,* 2013. *9*(8): p. 7796-805.

[142] Li Buay, K., et al., Epoxy Cross-Linked Collagen and Collagen-Laminin Peptide Hydrogels as Corneal Substitutes. *Journal of Functional Biomaterials, 2013. 4*(3): p. 162-77.

[143] Fagerholm, P., et al., Stable corneal regeneration four years after implantation of a cell-free recombinant human collagen scaffold. *Biomaterials,* 2014. *35*(8): p. 2420-2427.

[144] Builles, N., et al., Use of magnetically oriented orthogonal collagen scaffolds for hemi-corneal reconstruction and regeneration. *Biomaterials,* 2010. *31*(32): p. 8313-8322.

[145] Deng, C., et al., Collagen and glycopolymer based hydrogel for potential corneal application. *Acta Biomaterialia,* 2010. *6*(1): p. 187-194.

[146] Mi, S., et al., Photochemical cross-linking of plastically compressed collagen gel produces an optimal scaffold for corneal tissue engineering. *Journal of Biomedical Materials Research Part A,* 2011. *99A*(1): p. 1-8.

[147] Connon, C.J. and S. Mi, Photochemical cross-linking of plastically compressed collagen gel produces an improved and novel scaffold for corneal tissue engineering. *International Journal of Experimental Pathology,* 2011. *92*(6): p. A37-A37.

[148] Xiao, X., et al., In vivo study of the biocompatibility of a novel compressed collagen hydrogel scaffold for artificial corneas. *Journal of Biomedical Materials Research Part A,* 2014. *102*(6): p. 1782-1787.

[149] Li, X., et al., Morphologic Characteristics and Proliferation of Rabbit Corneal Stromal Cells Onto Complexes of Collagen-Chitosan-Sodium Hyaluronate Under Simulated Microgravity. *Investigative Ophthalmology & Visual Science,* 2013. *54*(10): p. 6877-6885.

[150] Giasson, C.J., et al., Adherens junction proteins are expressed in collagen corneal equivalents produced in vitro with human cells. *Molecular Vision,* 2014. *20*: p. 386-394.

[151] Naito, H., et al., Engineering bioartificial tracheal tissue using hybrid fibroblast-mesenchymal stem cell cultures in collagen hydrogels. *Interactive Cardiovascular and Thoracic Surgery*, 2011. *12*(2): p. 156-161.

[152] Dunphy, S.E., et al., Hydrogels for lung tissue engineering: Biomechanical properties of thin collagen-elastin constructs. *Journal of the Mechanical Behavior of Biomedical Materials,* 2014. *38*: p. 251-259.

[153] Zhao, Y., et al., In Vivo Generation of Thick, Vascularized Hepatic Tissue from Collagen Hydrogel-Based Hepatic Units. *Tissue Engineering Part C-Methods,* 2010. *16*(4): p. 653-659.

[154] Lee, J.H., et al., Collagen gel combined with mesoporous nanoparticles loading nerve growth factor as a feasible therapeutic three-dimensional depot for neural tissue engineering. *Rsc Advances,* 2013. *3*(46): p. 24202-24214.

[155] Martens, W., et al., Human dental pulp stem cells can differentiate into Schwann cells and promote and guide neurite outgrowth in an aligned tissue-engineered collagen construct in vitro. *Faseb Journal,* 2014. *28*(4): p. 1634-1643.

[156] Vonk, L.A., et al., Caprine articular, meniscus and intervertebral disc cartilage: An integral analysis of collagen network and chondrocytes. *Matrix Biology,* 2010. *29*(3): p. 209-218.

[157] Kwon, H., et al., The influence of scaffold material on chondrocytes under inflammatory conditions. *Acta Biomaterialia,* 2013. *9*(5): p. 6563-6575.

[158] Jones, D.G. and L. Peterson, Autologous chondrocyte implantation. *Journal of Bone and Joint Surgery-American Volume,* 2006. *88A*(11): p. 2502-2520.

[159] Harris, J.D., et al., Autologous Chondrocyte Implantation A Systematic Review. *Journal of Bone and Joint Surgery-American Volume,* 2010. *92A*(12): p. 2220-2233.

[160] Niemeyer, P., et al., Influence of Cell Quality on Clinical Outcome After Autologous Chondrocyte Implantation. *American Journal of Sports Medicine,* 2012. *40*(3): p. 556-561.

[161] Behery, O.A., et al., Factors Influencing the Outcome of Autologous Chondrocyte Implantation: A Systematic Review. *Journal of Knee Surgery,* 2013. *26*(3): p. 203-211.

[162] Peterson, L., et al., Autologous Chondrocyte Implantation A Long-term Follow-up. *American Journal of Sports Medicine*, 2010. *38*(6): p. 1117-1124.

[163] Pelissier, A., et al., Satisfactory long-term MRI after autologous chondrocyte implantation at the knee. *Knee Surgery Sports Traumatology Arthroscopy,* 2014. *22*(9): p. 2007-2012.

[164] Niemeyer, P., et al., Long-term Outcomes After First-Generation Autologous Chondrocyte Implantation for Cartilage Defects of the Knee. *American Journal of Sports Medicine,* 2014. *42*(1): p. 150-157.

[165] Ebert, J.R., et al., Clinical and Magnetic Resonance Imaging-Based Outcomes to 5 Years After Matrix-Induced Autologous Chondrocyte Implantation to Address Articular Cartilage Defects in the Knee. *American Journal of Sports Medicine,* 2011. *39*(4): p. 753-763.

[166] Ebert, J.R., et al., Correlation Between Clinical and Radiological Outcomes After Matrix-Induced Autologous Chondrocyte Implantation in the Femoral Condyles. *American Journal of Sports Medicine,* 2014. *42*(8): p. 1857-1864.

[167] Ebert, J.R., et al., Factors Predictive of Outcome 5 Years After Matrix-Induced Autologous Chondrocyte Implantation in the Tibiofemoral Joint. *American Journal of Sports Medicine,* 2013. *41*(6): p. 1245-1254.

[168] Enea, D., et al., Matrix-induced autologous chondrocyte implantation (MACI) in the knee. *Knee Surgery Sports Traumatology Arthroscopy,* 2012. *20*(5): p. 862-869.
[169] Meyerkort, D., et al., Matrix-induced autologous chondrocyte implantation (MACI) for chondral defects in the patellofemoral joint. *Knee Surgery Sports Traumatology Arthroscopy,* 2014. *22*(10): p. 2522-2530.
[170] Hindle, P., A.C. Hall, and L.C. Biant, Viability of Chondrocytes Seeded onto a Collagen I/III Membrane for Matrix-Induced Autologous Chondrocyte Implantation. *Journal of Orthopaedic Research,* 2014. *32*(11): p. 1495-1502.
[171] Schneider, U., et al., A Prospective Multicenter Study on the Outcome of Type I Collagen Hydrogel-Based Autologous Chondrocyte Implantation (CaReS) for the Repair of Articular Cartilage Defects in the Knee. *American Journal of Sports Medicine,* 2011. *39*(12): p. 2558-2565.
[172] Akgun, I., et al., Matrix-induced autologous mesenchymal stem cell implantation versus matrix-induced autologous chondrocyte implantation in the treatment of chondral defects of the knee: a 2-year randomized study. *Archives of Orthopaedic and Trauma Surgery,* 2015. *135*(2): p. 251-263.
[173] Edwards, P.K., et al., Arthroscopic Versus Open Matrix-Induced Autologous Chondrocyte Implantation: Results and Implications for Rehabilitation. *Journal of Sport Rehabilitation,* 2014. *23*(3): p. 203-215.
[174] Cai, Y., et al., Collagen grafted 3D polycaprolactone scaffolds for enhanced cartilage regeneration. *Journal of Materials Chemistry B,* 2013. *1*(43): p. 5971-5976.
[175] Chen, C.-H., et al., Selective laser sintered poly-epsilon-caprolactone scaffold hybridized with collagen hydrogel for cartilage tissue engineering. *Biofabrication,* 2014. *6*(1).
[176] Dai, W., et al., The influence of structural design of PLGA/collagen hybrid scaffolds in cartilage tissue engineering. *Biomaterials,* 2010. *31*(8): p. 2141-2152.
[177] Welsch, G.H., et al., Evaluation of Cartilage Repair Tissue After Matrix-Associated Autologous Chondrocyte Transplantation Using a Hyaluronic-Based or a Collagen-Based Scaffold With Morphological MOCART Scoring and Biochemical T2 Mapping Preliminary Results. *American Journal of Sports Medicine,* 2010. *38*(5): p. 934-942.

[178] Rutgers, M., et al., Effect of Collagen Type I or Type II on Chondrogenesis by Cultured Human Articular Chondrocytes. *Tissue Engineering Part A,* 2013. *19*(1-2): p. 59-65.

[179] Berendsen, A.D., et al., Contraction-induced Mmp13 and-14 expression by goat articular chondrocytes in collagen type I but not type II gels. *Journal of Tissue Engineering and Regenerative Medicine,* 2012. *6*(9): p. 721-730.

[180] Gavenis, K., et al., A Cell-Free Collagen Type I Device for the Treatment of Focal Cartilage Defects. *Artificial Organs,* 2010. *34*(1): p. 79-83.

[181] Mueller-Rath, R., et al., Condensed cellular seeded collagen gel as an improved biomaterial for tissue engineering of articular cartilage. *Bio-Medical Materials and Engineering,* 2010. *20*(6): p. 317-328.

[182] Puetzer, J.L. and L.J. Bonassar, High density type I collagen gels for tissue engineering of whole menisci. *Acta Biomaterialia,* 2013. *9*(8): p. 7787-7795.

[183] Makris, E.A., J.C. Hu, and K.A. Athanasiou, Hypoxia-induced collagen crosslinking as a mechanism for enhancing mechanical properties of engineered articular cartilage. *Osteoarthritis and Cartilage,* 2013. *21*(4): p. 634-641.

[184] Makris, E.A., et al., Developing functional musculoskeletal tissues through hypoxia and lysyl oxidase-induced collagen cross-linking. *Proceedings of the National Academy of Sciences of the United States of America,* 2014. *111*(45): p. E4832-E4841.

[185] Deponti, D., et al., Collagen Scaffold for Cartilage Tissue Engineering: The Benefit of Fibrin Glue and the Proper Culture Time in an Infant Cartilage Model. *Tissue Engineering Part A,* 2014. *20*(5-6): p. 1113-1126.

[186] Yang, Y.-H., et al., Type I Collagen-Based Fibrous Capsule Enhances Integration of Tissue-Engineered Cartilage with Native Articular Cartilage. *Annals of Biomedical Engineering,* 2014. *42*(4): p. 716-726.

[187] Chicatun, F., et al., Effect of Chitosan Incorporation and Scaffold Geometry on Chondrocyte Function in Dense Collagen Type I Hydrogels. *Tissue Engineering Part A,* 2013. *19*(23-24): p. 2553-2564.

[188] Guo, Y., et al., Hydrogels of collagen/chondroitin sulfate/hyaluronan interpenetrating polymer network for cartilage tissue engineering. *Journal of Materials Science-Materials in Medicine,* 2012. *23*(9): p. 2267-2279.

[189] Li, Y., et al., The Effects of Insulin-Like Growth Factor-1 and Basic Fibroblast Growth Factor on the Proliferation of Chondrocytes Embedded in the Collagen Gel Using an Integrated Microfluidic Device. *Tissue Engineering Part C-Methods,* 2010. *16*(6): p. 1267-1275.
[190] Rosenzweig, D.H., et al., Cartilaginous constructs using primary chondrocytes from continuous expansion culture seeded in dense collagen gels. *Acta Biomaterialia,* 2013. *9*(12): p. 9360-9369.
[191] Nebelung, S., et al., Continuous cyclic compressive loading modulates biological and mechanical properties of collagen hydrogels seeded with human chondrocytes. *Biorheology, 2011. 48*(5-6): p. 247-261.
[192] Nebelung, S., et al., Simultaneous anabolic and catabolic responses of human chondrocytes seeded in collagen hydrogels to long-term continuous dynamic compression. *Annals of Anatomy-Anatomischer Anzeiger,* 2012. *194*(4): p. 351-358.
[193] Zhang, X.J., et al., The effect of non-growth factors on chondrogenic differentiation of mesenchymal stem cells. *Cell and Tissue Banking,* 2014. *15*(3): p. 319-327.
[194] Zheng, L., et al., Chondrogenic differentiation of mesenchymal stem cells induced by collagen-based hydrogel: An in vivo study. *Journal of Biomedical Materials Research Part A,* 2010. *93A*(2): p. 783-792.
[195] Zhang, L., et al., An in vitro study of collagen hydrogel to induce the chondrogenic differentiation of mesenchymal stem cells. *Journal of Biomedical Materials Research Part A,* 2012. *100A*(10): p. 2717-2725.
[196] Zheng, L., et al., Material-induced chondrogenic differentiation of mesenchymal stem cells is material-dependent. *Experimental and Therapeutic Medicine,* 2014. *7*(5): p. 1147-1150.
[197] Meng, F., et al., Chondrogenic differentiation of ATDC5 and hMSCs could be induced by a novel scaffold-tricalcium phosphate-collagen-hyaluronan without any exogenous growth factors in vitro. *Journal of Biomedical Materials Research Part A,* 2014. *102*(8): p. 2725-2735.
[198] Chen, X., et al., Chondrogenic differentiation of umbilical cord-derived mesenchymal stem cells in type I collagen-hydrogel for cartilage engineering. *Injury-International Journal of the Care of the Injured,* 2013. *44*(4): p. 540-549.
[199] Dinescu, S., et al., Biocompatibility Assessment of Novel Collagen-Sericin Scaffolds Improved with Hyaluronic Acid and Chondroitin Sulfate for Cartilage Regeneration. *BioMed research international,* 2013: p. 1-11.

[200] Damaraju, S., et al., The Effect of Mechanical Stimulation on Mineralization in Differentiating Osteoblasts in Collagen-I Scaffolds. *Tissue Engineering Part A, 2014. 20*(23-24): p. 3142-3153.

[201] Zhang, S., et al., Bi-layer collagen/microporous electrospun nanofiber scaffold improves the osteochondral regeneration. *Acta Biomaterialia,* 2013. *9*(7): p. 7236-7247.

[202] Zhang, W., et al., The promotion of osteochondral repair by combined intra-articular injection of parathyroid hormone-related protein and implantation of a bi-layer collagen-silk scaffold. *Biomaterials,* 2013. *34*(25): p. 6046-6057.

[203] Chen, P., et al., Radially oriented collagen scaffold with SDF-1 promotes osteochondral repair by facilitating cell homing. *Biomaterials,* 2015. *39*: p. 114-23.

[204] Zhou, J., et al., In vitro generation of osteochondral differentiation of human marrow mesenchymal stem cells in novel collagen-hydroxyapatite layered scaffolds. *Acta Biomaterialia,* 2011. *7*(11): p. 3999-4006.

[205] Maehara, H., et al., Repair of Large Osteochondral Defects in Rabbits Using Porous Hydroxyapatite/Collagen (HAp/Col) and Fibroblast Growth Factor-2 (FGF-2). *Journal of Orthopaedic Research,* 2010. *28*(5): p. 677-686.

[206] Zheng, L., et al., Evaluation of novel in situ synthesized nano-hydroxyapatite/collagen/alginate hydrogels for osteochondral tissue engineering. *Biomedical Materials,* 2014. *9*(6).

[207] Orgel, J.P., J.D. San Antonio, and O. Antipova, Molecular and structural mapping of collagen fibril interactions. *Connect Tissue Res,* 2011. *52*(1): p. 2-17.

[208] Leikina, E., et al., Type I collagen is thermally unstable at body temperature. *Proceedings of the National Academy of Sciences of the United States of America,* 2002. *99*(3): p. 1314-1318.

[209] Orgel, J.P.R.O., et al., Microfibrillar structure of type I collagen in situ. *Proceedings of the National Academy of Sciences of the United States of America,* 2006. *103*(24): p. 9001-9005.

[210] Okuyama, K., et al., Comment on Microfibrillar structure of type I collagen in situ by Orgel et al. (2006), Proc. Natl Acad. Sci. USA, 103, 9001-9005. *Acta Crystallographica Section D-Biological Crystallography,* 2009. *65*: p. 1007-1008.

[211] Orgel, J.P.R.O., On the packing structure of collagen: response to Okuyama et al.'s comment on Microfibrillar structure of type I collagen

in situ. *Acta Crystallographica Section D-Biological Crystallography,* 2009. *65*: p. 1009-1010.

[212] Orgel, J.P., et al., Collagen fibril surface displays a constellation of sites capable of promoting fibril assembly, stability, and hemostasis. *Connect Tissue Res,* 2011. *52*(1): p. 18-24.

[213] Orgel, J.P., A.V. Persikov, and O. Antipova, Variation in the helical structure of native collagen. *Plos One,* 2014. *9*(2): p. e89519.

[214] Chen, X., et al., Second harmonic generation microscopy for quantitative analysis of collagen fibrillar structure. *Nat Protoc,* 2012. *7*(4): p. 654-69.

[215] Cicchi, R., et al., From molecular structure to tissue architecture: collagen organization probed by SHG microscopy. *J Biophotonics,* 2013. *6*(2): p. 129-42.

[216] Mercado, K.P., et al., Characterizing collagen microstructure using high frequency ultrasound. *The Journal of the Acoustical Society of America,* 2014. *135*(4): p. 2373-2373.

[217] Wallace, J.M., et al., Type I Collagen Exists as a Distribution of Nanoscale Morphologies in Teeth, Bones, and Tendons. *Langmuir,* 2010. *26*(10): p. 7349-7354.

[218] Fang, M., et al., Type I Collagen D-Spacing in Fibril Bundles of Dermis, Tendon, and Bone: Bridging between Nano- and Micro-Level Tissue Hierarchy. *Acs Nano,* 2012. *6*(11): p. 9503-9514.

[219] Erickson, B., et al., Nanoscale structure of type I collagen fibrils: quantitative measurement of D-spacing. *Biotechnol J,* 2013. *8*(1): p. 117-26.

[220] Su, H.N., et al., The ultrastructure of type I collagen at nanoscale: large or small D-spacing distribution? *Nanoscale,* 2014. *6*(14): p. 8134-8139.

[221] Wallace, J.M., Comment on "The ultrastructure of type I collagen at nanoscale: large or small D-spacing distribution?" by H.-N. Su, L.-Y. Ran, Z.-H. Chen, Q.-L. Qin, M. Shi, X.-Y. Song, X.-L. Chen, Y.-Z. Zhang and B.-B. Xie, Nanoscale, 2014, 6, 8134. *Nanoscale,* 2015. *7*(3): p. 1233-1234.

[222] Su, H.N. and B.B. Xie, Reply to the comment on "The ultrastructure of type I collagen at nanoscale: large or small D-spacing distribution?" by J. Wallace, Nanoscale, 2015, 7, DOI: 10.1039/c4nr03160a. *Nanoscale,* 2015. *7*(3): p. 1235-1236.

[223] Israelowitz, M., et al., Computational modeling of type I collagen fibers to determine the extracellular matrix structure of connective tissues. *Protein Eng Des Sel,* 2005. *18*(7): p. 329-35.

[224] Brown, E.M., Development and utilization of a bovine type I collagen microfibril model. *Int J Biol Macromol,* 2013. *53*: p. 20-5.

[225] Soares, A.L.F., C.W.J. Oomens, and F.P.T. Baaijens, A computational model to describe the collagen orientation in statically cultured engineered tissues. *Computer Methods in Biomechanics and Biomedical Engineering,* 2014. *17*(3): p. 251-262.

[226] Silva, T.H., et al., Marine Origin Collagens and Its Potential Applications. *Marine Drugs,* 2014. *12*(12): p. 5881-5901.

[227] Yamada, S., et al., Potency of Fish Collagen as a Scaffold for Regenerative Medicine. *Biomed Research International,* 2014.

[228] Fernandes-Silva, S., et al., Porous Hydrogels From Shark Skin Collagen Crosslinked Under Dense Carbon Dioxide Atmosphere. *Macromolecular Bioscience,* 2013. *13*(11): p. 1621-1631.

[229] Di Benedetto, C., et al., Production, Characterization and Biocompatibility of Marine Collagen Matrices from an Alternative and Sustainable Source: The Sea Urchin Paracentrotus lividus. *Marine Drugs,* 2014. *12*(9): p. 4912-4933.

[230] Ramanathan, G., et al., Extraction and Characterization of Collagen from the Skin of Arothron stellatus Fish-A Novel Source of Collagen for Tissue Engineering. *Journal of Biomaterials and Tissue Engineering,* 2014. *4*(3): p. 203-209.

[231] Lin, Z., et al., In vitro Evaluation of Natural Marine Sponge Collagen as a Scaffold for Bone Tissue Engineering. *International Journal of Biological Sciences, 2011*. *7*(7): p. 968-977.

[232] Krishnan, S., et al., Fish Scale Collagen-A Novel Material for Corneal Tissue Engineering. *Artificial Organs,* 2012. *36*(9): p. 829-835.

[233] Pallela, R., et al., Biophysicochemical evaluation of chitosan-hydroxyapatite-marine sponge collagen composite for bone tissue engineering. *Journal of Biomedical Materials Research Part A,* 2012. *100A*(2): p. 486-495.

[234] Bermueller, C., et al., Marine Collagen Scaffolds for Nasal Cartilage Repair: Prevention of Nasal Septal Perforations in a New Orthotopic Rat Model Using Tissue Engineering Techniques. *Tissue Engineering Part A*, 2013. *19*(19-20): p. 2201-2214.

[235] Hoyer, B., et al., Jellyfish collagen scaffolds for cartilage tissue engineering. *Acta Biomaterialia,* 2014. *10*(2): p. 883-892.

[236] Ruggiero, F., et al., Triple helix assembly and processing of human collagen produced in transgenic tobacco plants. *Febs Letters,* 2000. *469*(1): p. 132-136.

[237] Shoseyov, O., Y. Posen, and F. Grynspan, Human Recombinant Type I Collagen Produced in Plants. *Tissue Engineering Part A,* 2013. *19*(13-14): p. 1527-1533.

[238] Shoseyov, O., Y. Posen, and F. Grynspan, Human collagen produced in plants More than just another molecule. *Bioengineered,* 2014. *5*(1): p. 49-52.

[239] Willard, J.J., et al., Plant-Derived Human Collagen Scaffolds for Skin Tissue Engineering. *Tissue Engineering Part A,* 2013. *19*(13-14): p. 1507-1518.

[240] Yu, S.M., Y. Li, and D. Kim, Collagen mimetic peptides: progress towards functional applications. *Soft Matter,* 2011. *7*(18): p. 7927-7938.

[241] Li, Y. and S.M. Yu, Targeting and mimicking collagens via triple helical peptide assembly. *Current Opinion in Chemical Biology,* 2013. *17*(6): p. 968-975.

[242] He, L.R. and P. Theato, Collagen and collagen mimetic peptide conjugates in polymer science. *European Polymer Journal,* 2013. *49*(10): p. 2986-2997.

[243] Lee, H.J., et al., Collagen mimetic peptide-conjugated photopolymerizable PEG hydrogel. *Biomaterials,* 2006. *27*(30): p. 5268-5276.

[244] Li, Y., et al., Direct Detection of Collagenous Proteins by Fluorescently Labeled Collagen Mimetic Peptides. *Bioconjugate Chemistry,* 2013. *24*(1): p. 9-16.

[245] Santos, J.L., et al., Conducting polymer nanoparticles decorated with collagen mimetic peptides for collagen targeting. *Chemical Communications,* 2014. *50*(95): p. 15045-15048.

[246] Krishnamoorthy, N., M.H. Yacoub, and S.N. Yaliraki, A computational modeling approach for enhancing self-assembly and biofunctionalisation of collagen biomimetic peptides. *Biomaterials,* 2011. *32*(30): p. 7275-7285.

[247] Sarkar, B., L.E.R. O'Leary, and J.D. Hartgerink, Self-Assembly of Fiber-Forming Collagen Mimetic Peptides Controlled by Triple-Helical Nucleation. *Journal of the American Chemical Society,* 2014. *136*(41): p. 14417-14424.

In: Type I Collagen
Editor: Gretchen Rivera

ISBN: 978-1-63482-829-1

Chapter 2

Structural Analyses of Type I Collagen Fibrils for Application to Tissue Engineering

Koichi Morimoto [*] ***and Saori Kunii***
Department of Genetic Engineering, Kindai University,
Nishimitani, Kinokawa, Wakayama, Japan

Abstract

Type I collagen molecules spontaneously form insoluble fibrils at physiological buffers and at neutral pH. Insoluble fibrils play an important role in not only structure stabilization in tissue but also maintenance of each cell. Recently, collagen has been used as one of cell scaffolds in regenerative medicine. In cell culture conditions, the structure of molecule in collagen fibrils would be different from that of collagen monomer. Then, the study in ultrastructure of fibril is more important than that of monomer to understand cell behaviors. However, the structural information is not well understood yet. In this Chapter, we report on the helicity of collagen molecule in fibrils by circular dichroism spectroscopy and the thermograph of fibrils by differential scanning calorimetry. Furthermore, we observed the appearance of mouse

[*] Koichi Morimoto, Department of Genetic Engineering, Kindai University, 930 Nishimitani, Kinokawa, Wakayama 649-6493, Japan. Tel.: +81-736-77-3888; Fax: +81-736-77-4754; E-mail: morimoto@waka.kindai.ac.jp

neutrophil on collagen scaffolds showing imperfect fibrils. Our data indicated that the ultrastructure of collagen molecule depends on monomer or fibrils. We suggest that the formation of collagen fibrils prior to cell seeding is necessary for the interaction between cells and extracellular matrices.

Introduction

Type I collagen is the most abundant protein in connective tissues such as skin, bone, tendon, and ligaments. Each collagen molecule contains N-telopeptide, triple-helical, and C-telopeptide domains [1], and at physiological conditions the molecules spontaneously assemble into a fibrous structure. To precisely elucidate the conformation of the collagen molecule and its thermal stability, numerous collagens and collagen-like model peptides have been studied. In addition, a number of models have been proposed to describe the self-assembly of ordered fibrils [2–8]. The most important event during fibrillogenesis is the lateral association between collagen helices. Packing of collagen molecules into fibrils is thought to affect physiological functions, such as proliferation, differentiation, adhesion, and hemostasis [9–14]. These fibrils are insoluble, and resistant to proteinases, and provide mechanical strength and integrity to the body. Based on scanning electron microscopy (SEM) and atomic force microscopy (AFM), the surface of this fibril shows a D-staggered arrangement with a unit length of 67 nm [15,16], and lateral packing of adjacent collagen molecules results in a quasi-hexagonal structure. Quasi-hexagonal lateral packing reveals the characteristic aspects of the surface of these fibrils [12]. Local fluctuations in collagen conformation may alter accessibility to the surface of the collagen fibril and affect binding to macromolecular partners [17, 18]. However, very little is known about intermolecular interactions between side chains of collagen helices during self-association. For the first line of defense against the pathogens, neutrophils migrate into the tissue infected with bacteria. Therefore, the rapid response of neutrophils in the extracellular matrix is the most important immunological event. In our body, neutrophils actively invade into collagen fibrils to seek pathogens. Activated neutrophils have a highly convoluted cell membrane that forms protruding pseudopods [19]. Probably, neutrophils alter themselves by the extracellular microenvironments. To precisely understand the function, it is necessary to investigate in a brief period in vitro. However, the morphological change of neutrophils in collagen fibrils still remains to be clarified.

To study the structure and function of collagen in vitro many researchers have used pepsin-hydrolyzed collagen (Pep-Col) [8, 17, 18, 20–22], which spontaneously forms fibril with the D-periodic staggered pattern in vitro [23, 24]. To clarify the superstructure of collagen used as a scaffold for cell culture, we characterized the time dependence of self-assembly kinetics by using conventional turbidity measurements and circular dichroism (CD) measurements. Also, we used CD to assess the triple-helical content of self-assembled Pep-Col fibrils. Thermal stability of Pep-Col self-assembly was measured using differential scanning calorimetry (DSC) (pH range 4.0–7.3) and by obtaining transition temperatures and calorimetric enthalpies. The appearances of neutrophil's membrane surface and collagen self-assembly were observed by ultra-high resolution SEM.

Materials and Methods

Preparation of Pep-Col

Acid-soluble type I collagen was extracted from chicken skin. Pep-Col was prepared as described [25, 26]. Collagen concentrations were determined by weighing lyophilized preparations. The molecular weight of Pep-Col was estimated to be 275×10^3, based on amino-acid composition (UniProtKB/Swiss-Prot database: COL1A1, ver. 92; and COL1A2, ver. 104).

Turbidity Measurements

Self-assembly kinetics for Pep-Col was estimated by measuring turbidity changes at 313 nm using a MultiSpec-1500 spectrophotometer (Shimadzu Corporation, Kyoto, Japan). Pep-Col was dissolved in 20 mM sodium acetate buffer (pH 4.0) to a final concentration of 10 mg/ml. Pep-Col solution was then diluted to 0.20 mg/ml with 40 mM sodium phosphate buffer (pH 5.8 or 7.3). Prior to measuring turbidity, each collagen solution was incubated in a capillary cell for 30 min at 25°C. The temperature was then increased to 35°C and the measurements were initiated. The following parameters were estimated manually from the turbidity curve: the maximum absorbance at 313 nm (ΔA_{313}), the maximum fibril growth rate ($(\mathrm{d}A/\mathrm{d}t)_{max}$), and the time at which the maximum fibril growth rate was observed (t_{max}) [25].

DSC Measurements

Thermal denaturation curves were constructed using the Nano DSC differential scanning calorimeter (Calorimetry Sciences Corporation, Lindon, UT). Measurements were taken from 35°C to 70°C using 0.895-ml gold capillary cells [27]. Each thermogram was corrected by subtracting values obtained using a buffer control. A constant heating rate of 1.0°C/min was used. To obtain the thermodynamic equilibrium state of self-assembled Pep-Col, solutions were pre-incubated at 35°C for 120 min. The transition temperature (T_m) and calorimetric enthalpy change (ΔH) were determined from the melting-peak maximum and the melting-peak area, respectively. These thermodynamic parameters were calculated using NanoAnalyze software version 2.2.0 (TA Instruments, New Castle, DE). Measurements concerning pH dependence were carried out using collagen preparations (0.20 mg/ml) in 40 mM sodium acetate buffer (pH 4.0) or 40 mM sodium phosphate buffer (pH 5.8 and pH 7.3). The molecular weight of Pep-Col is 275×10^3.

CD Spectroscopy

CD measurements were performed using a J-820 spectropolarimeter (JASCO Corporation, Tokyo, Japan) with a Perche temperature controller (JASCO). Measurements were taken from 250–190 nm using a 1-mm cell. Pep-Col (0.20 mg/ml) was dissolved in 40 mM sodium phosphate buffer (pH 7.3) at 20°C. Before measurements of the incubation time dependence were taken, Pep-Col solutions were incubated in measurement cells for 10, 90, or 120 min at 35°C. Melting curves (10–70°C) at pH 4.0 and pH 7.3 were measured at 220 nm with the heating rate of 1°C/min. The melting temperature obtained by CD measurements indicates as T_d. For all collagen preparations, CD was measured at <600 V.

Scanning Electron Microscopy of Neutrophil on Pep-Col

To investigate neutrophil's morphology and Pep-Col fibrillogenesis, we observed cell surface and imperfect fibrils with an S-900 ultra-high resolution scanning electron microscope (HITACHI, Tokyo, Japan) with an accelerating voltage of 10 kV. Three glass disks (13 mm diameter) were coated with Pep-Col solution (3 mg/mL) in 15 mM acetic acid and air-dried at 20°C. Then, each glass disk was inserted into a well of 24 well culture plate. Subsequently, freshly isolated mouse neutrophils suspended in 10% FBS DMEM were carefully added into the well. After an incubation period of 3, 60, or 120 min, each glass disk was placed in 2% glutaraldehyde solution at room temperature for 1 h. Sample preparation for SEM observation were carried out according to the methods of Nakayama et al. [28].

Results

Turbidity Increasing by Self-assembly Formation

Turbidity measurements were carried out to determine the incubation time, necessary to reach the plateau phase at pH 5.8 and pH 7.3. The turbidity progress curves (Figure 1) show that the kinetics of self-assembly formation of Pep-Col drastically depended on pH. The t_{max}, $(dA/dt)_{max}$, and A_{313} are summarized in Table 1. Pep-Col molecules have formed self-assembly before 180 min under the observed pHs. Therefore, in other experiments, the end-point time of Pep-Col self-assembly formation was set for 120 min.

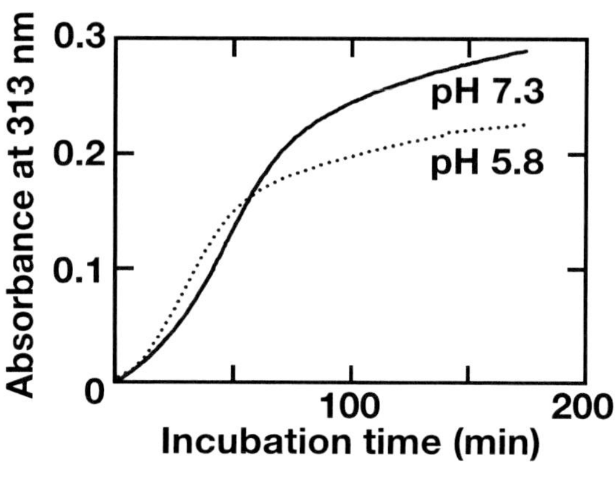

Figure 1. Effect of pH on the self-assembly of Pep-Col as monitored by turbidity increase at 35°C. Turbidity was measured at 313 nm in 40 mM phosphate buffer. The concentration of Pep-Col was 0.2 mg/mL, and each incubation time was 180 min. Dashed line and solid line indicate the turbidity curve at pH 5.8 and at pH 7.3, respectively.

Table 1. Kinetic parameters of pep-Col self-assembly at pH 5.8. and pH 7.3

pH	ΔA_{313}	$(dA/dt)_{max} \cdot 10^2$ (A_{313}/min)	t_{max} (min)
5.8	0.234	0.546	27
7.3	0.306	0.558	40

Thermal Stability of Pep-Col

We planned to obtain thermograms of collagen self-assembly by DSC from 35°C to 70°C under the equilibrium conditions. In order to achieve the equilibrium state of self-assembly formation, Pep-Col solution was kept in the capillary cell for 120 min at 35°C, prior to measurements.

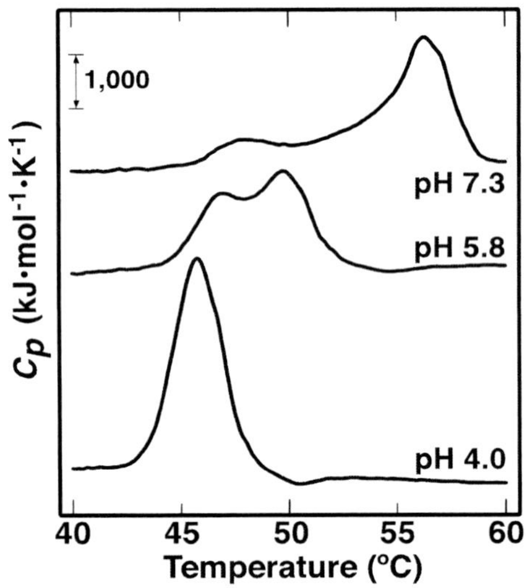

Figure 2. Effect of pH on DSC thermogram of Pep-Col. Measurements were taken between 35°C and 70°C using a heating rate of 1.0°C/min. Data from 40°C to 60°C are shown. Before the DSC thermograms were generated, each Pep-Col solution (0.20 mg/ml) was pre-incubated in the capillary cell for 120 min at 35°C. The buffer solution was 40 mM sodium acetate (pH 4.0) or 40 mM sodium phosphate (pH 5.8 and 7.3) The T_m is the temperature of the apparent maximum peak, and ΔH_{cal} is the calorimetric enthalpy change of the total peak.

The effects of pH on DSC thermogram were shown in Figure 2. The highest temperature at C_p value (T_m) and the ΔH_{cal} of thermogram were determined by a NanoAnalyze software and shown in Table 2. The thermogram profile at pH 5.8 was exhibited apparent two distinct peaks at 46.9°C and 49.6°C, whereas the peak at pH 4.0 and pH 7.3 showed around 45.7°C and 56.3°C, respectively (Figure 2). Thus, the thermal stability of self-assembly at neutral pH was shown to increase by the self-assembly formation. Probably, the thermograms at pH 4.0 would indicate the transition pathway from the monomeric structure to the disordered structure. The ΔH_{cal} values of Pep-Col were similar between pH 4.0 and pH 7.3 (Table 2).

Table 2. T_m and ΔHcal of Pep-Col self-assembly at pH 4.0, pH 5.8. and pH 7.3

pH	T_m (°C)	ΔH_{cal} (kJ•mol^{-1})
4.0	45.7	11.400
5.8	49.6	9.400
7.3	56.3	11.900

Circular Dichroism Spectroscopy of Pep-Col Self-assemblies

A collagen molecule exhibits the typical CD spectrum of the triple-helix in the range 190–250 nm as our previous reports [25, 26]. We tried to measure the changes of CD spectrum upon collagen self-assembly formation at 35°C and pH 7.3, in spite of the fact that the turbidity was high under these conditions.

Figure 3 shows that the positive peak at 220 nm of Pep-Col slightly but markedly decreased within 10 min at 35°C. As the incubation-time progressed, the peak top of Pep-Col slightly red-shifted from 220 nm (Figure 3). The melting curve at pH 7.3 indicated that Pep-Col forms fibril during heating from 28°C to 43°C (Figure 4). The T_d of Pep-Col self-assembly at pH 4.0 and pH 7.3 was 42.7°C and 52.0°C, respectively. These T_d values were lower than T_m values obtained by the thermogram measurements.

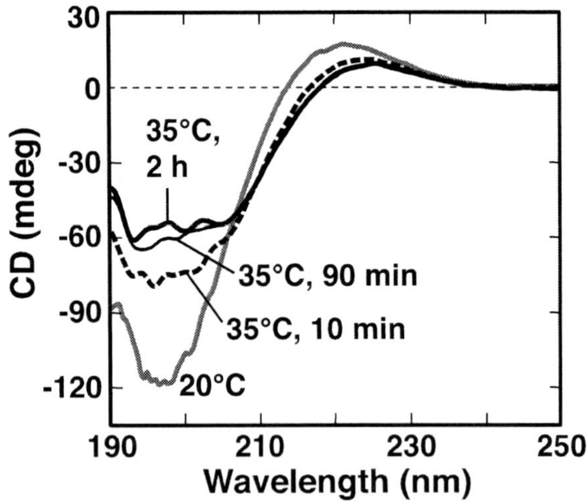

Figure 3. Time-dependence of CD spectra of Pep-Col. All measurements were performed in a 1-mm cell controlled by a Perche system. The Pep-Col concentration was 0.20 mg/mL in 40 mM phosphate buffer, pH 7.3. CD spectrum was measured from 190 to 250 nm after pre-incubation for 10 min, 90 min, or 120 min at 35°C. As a reference, CD spectrum of Pep-Col at 20°C was measured.

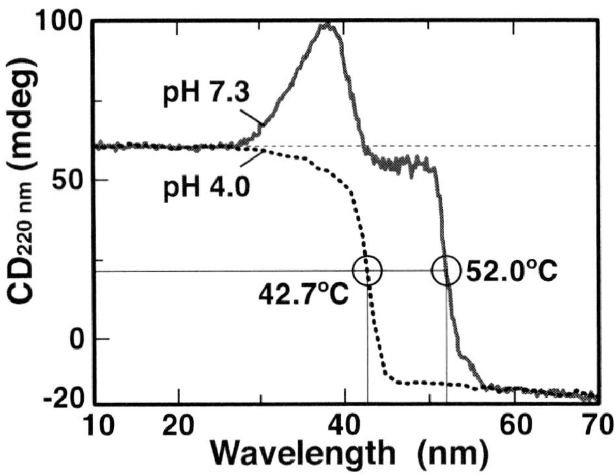

Figure 4. Melting curve of Pep-Col by CD measurements. The concentration of Pep-Col preparation was 0.20 mg/mL. The CD value was monitored at 220 nm from 10°C to 70°C. Dashed line and solid line indicate the melting curve at pH 4.0 and at pH 7.3, respectively. Each T_d was estimated from the melting curve (open circle).

Scanning Electron Microscopy (SEM) of Neutrophil on Pep-Col

To further elucidate the difference of the structure of Pep-Col fibrils, we inspected the scanning electron micrographs of Pep-Col self-assemblies formed under the conditions of 3, 60, or 120 min incubation in 10% FBS DMEM at pH 7.2-7.4 (Figure 5). Moreover, the morphology of neutrophils on Pep-Col matrices was also observed at the same time. In the culture medium, Pep-Col coated on a plastic culture dish formed self-assembly depending on incubation time from 3 min to 120 min. As shown in Figure 5A and 5B, the microspike on the cell surface of neutrophil was highly complex with the imperfect Pep-Col fibrils. However, after 120 min incubation, Pep-Col showed thin microfibril structure and a D-periodic banding pattern (white arrow in Figure 5C), and the cell surface of neutrophil changed into larger protrusions (black arrow in Figure 5C).

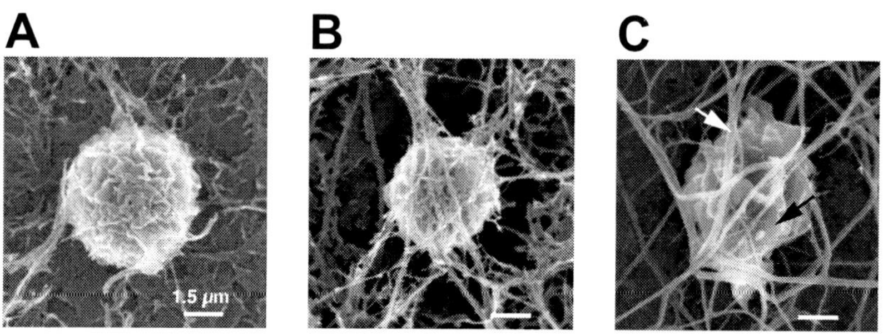

Figure 5. SEM micrographs of neutrophils on Pep-Col incubated at pH 7.3. Neutrophils were incubated at 37°C for 3 min (A), 60 min (B), or 120 min (C). From the same time of cell seeding, Pep-Col molecules slowly began to form fibrils. The black arrow indicates protrusion of membrane surface and white arrow indicates Pep-Col self-assembly.

Discussion

The kinetic parameters of self-assembly formation at pH 5.8 and pH 7.3 were obtained by measuring the turbidity increasing. There is no evidence for that the suprastructures of the self-assembly in plateau phase (ΔA_{313}) were similar (Figure 1). The structure of each self-assembly must be different from others and will be revealed by analyzing the thermal stability.

To better distinguish between the collagen molecule and collagen self-assembly, we investigated the thermal stability of the collagen self-assembly by conventional DSC at pH 4.0 pH 5.8, or pH 7.3. In each measurement, collagen concentration was set for 0.20 mg/mL (Figure 2). The T_m peak at pH 4.0 indicates the melting of triple-helical structure of monomeric collagen molecule [29]. On the other hand, that at pH 7.3 shows the melting of triple-helical structure in collagen self-assembly. The T_m of Pep-Col self-assembly, at pH 4.0 and pH 7.3, was 46.9°C and 56.3°C, respectively. There is a drastic change in the thermogram profile of between pH 4.0 and pH 7.3 (Figure 2). Interestingly, the thermogram profile at pH 5.8 showed clearly distinct two peaks. It might mean the initial stage of collagen fibrillogenesis including both molecules and microfibrils. Probably, pH 5.8 is the most important pH to change the electrostatic charges on the surface of collagen molecule to progress to self-assembly.

The ratio of CD positive peak intensity over CD negative peak intensity, R_{pn}, represents an index for triple-helical structure of collagen molecule [30]. In our experiments, the R_{pn} value of Pep-Col increased from 0.136 to 0.158 during 120 min incubation at 35°C at pH 7.3 (Figure 3). The increase of the R_{pn} value means an increase of the helicity and, in turn, an increase in thermal stability. The time-dependence of CD spectrum (Figure 3) and that of turbidity curve (Figure 1) of Pep-Col were almost similar each other in time scale. Therefore, we hypothesize that the self-assembly formation would involve the conformation change from "looser-packing form" to "tight form". The existence of looser and tighter regions within the triple-helical domain is commonly accepted.

The T_d determined by CD melting curve (Figure 4) was inconsistent with the T_m by DSC thermogram (Figure 2). The T_m value at pH 4.0 was 45.7°C, and the T_d value was 42.7°C. At pH 7.3, the T_m value was 56.3°C and the T_d was 52.0°C. This discrepancy can be explained by the principal of each measurement. The collapse of triple-helical structure would be detected earlier than the denaturation of tertiary structure.

The SEM micrographs of neutrophil on Pep-Col have provided a visualization of time dependence of neutrophil's morphology and fibril formation (Figure 5). Pep-Col coated on a culture dish needs the pre-incubation for 120 min at least at 37°C to form the self-assembly. This result is consistent with the turbidity curve (Figure 1) and the thermogram (Figure 2). Interestingly, the appearance of neutrophil seemed to clearly change between 3 min and 120 min (Figure 5).

We found direct evidence that the helicity of collagen during an incubation period increase to assemble spontaneously and that they enhance the thermal stability at neutral pH. In the cell culture, the coated collagen needs 120 min incubation at least at 37°C to perfectly form fibrils before cell seeding. It is a very important process for the investigation of the interaction between cells and matrices.

Acknowledgments

Authors are grateful to Professor Takuya Saito and Ms Michiko Shibano of Kindai University for expert technical assistance of scanning electron microscopy. We deeply thank Professor Ben'ichiro Tonomura of Kindai University and Professor Harumi Fukada of Osaka Prefecture University for valuable discussions.

Abbreviations

CD, circular dichroism;
DMEM, Dulbecco's modified Eagle medium;
DSC, differential scanning calorimetry;
FBS, fetal bovine serum;
Pep-Col, pepsin-hydrolyzed collagen;
SEM, scanning electron microscopy.

References

[1] Veis, A., and George, A. (1994) *Extracellular Matrix Assembly and Structure* (Yurchenco, P. D., Birk, D. E., and Mechanm, R. P., eds.) 1st Ed., Academic Press, Inc., San Diego, CA, 15–45.

[2] Inouye, K., Kobayashi, Y., Kyogoku, Y., Kishida, Y., Sakakibara, S., and Prockop, D.J. (1982) *Arch. Biochem. Biophys.* 219, 198–203.

[3] Miles, C.A., Burjanadze, T.V., and Bailey, A.J. (1995) *J. Mol. Biol.* 245, 437–446.

[4] Kramer, R.Z., Bella, J., Mayville, P., Brodsky, B., and Berman, H. M. (1999) *Nature Structural Biology* 6, 454–457.

[5] Jiravanichanun, N., Hongo, C., Wu, G., Noguchi, K., Okuyama, K., and Nishino, N.T. (2005) *ChemBioChem* 6, 1184–1187.
[6] Orgel, J.P.R.O., Irving, T.C., Miller, A., and Wess, T.J. (2006) *PNAS* 103, 9001–9005.
[7] Mu, C., Li, D., Lin, W., Ding, Y., and Zhang, G. (2007) *Biopolymers* 86, 282–287.
[8] Berisio, R., DeSimone, A., Ruggiero, A., Improta, R., and Vitagliano L. (2008) *J. Pept. Sci.* 15, 131–140.
[9] Holmes, D.F., Gilpin, C.J., Baldock, C., Ziese, U., Koster, A.J., and Kadler, K.E. (2001) *PNAS* 98, 7307–7312.
[10] Stoop, R., Kotani, H., McNeish, J. D., Otterness, I. G., and Mikecz, K. (2001) *Arthritis Rheum.* 44, 2922–2931.
[11] Smethurst, P.A., Onley, D.J., Jarvis, G.E., O'Connor, M.N., Knight, C.G., Herr, A.B., Ouwehand, W.H., and Farndale, R.W. (2007) *J. Biol. Chem.* 282, 1296–1304.
[12] Sweeney, S.M., Orgel, J.P., Fertala, A., McAuliffe, J.D., Turner, K.R., Di Lullo, G.A., Chen, S., Antipova, O., Perumal, S., Ala-Kokko, L., Forlino, A., Cabral, W.A., Barnes, A.M., Marini, J.C., and San Antonio, J.D. (2008) *J. Biol. Chem.* 283, 21187–21197.
[13] Rygiel, T.P., Stolte, E.H., de Ruiter, T., van de Weijer, M.L., Meyaard, L. (2011) *Mol. Immunol.* 49, 402–406.
[14] Ruiz, P.A., and Jarai, G. (2012) *Fibrogenesis Tissue Repair* 5, 3–9.
[15] Morimoto, K., Kawabata, K. Kunii, S., Hamano, K., Saito, T., and Tonomura, B. (2009) *J. Biochem.* 145, 677–684.
[16] Paige, M.F., Rainey, J.K., and Goh, M.C. (1998) *Biophys. J.* 74, 3211–3216.
[17] Perumal, S., Antipova, O., and Orgel, J.P.R.O. (2008) *PNAS* 105, 2824–2829.
[18] Orgel, J.P.R.O., Antipova, O., Sagi, I., Bitler, A., Qiu, D., Wang, R., Xu, Y., and Antonio, J.D., (2011) *Connect. Tissue Res.* 52, 18–24.
[19] Paape, M. J., Banneman, D. D., Zhao, X., and Lee, J. W. (2003) *Vet. Res.* 34, 597–627.
[20] 20. Brennan, M., and Davison P.F. (1981) *Biopolymers* 20, 2195–2202.
[21] Villarreal, F., Omens, J., Dillmann, W., Risteli, J., Nguyen, J., and Covell, J. (2004) *J. Mol. Cell. Card.* 36, 597–601.
[22] 22. Malone, J. P., and Veis, A. (2004) *Biochemistry* 43, 15358–15366.
[23] 23. Capaldi, M.J., and Chapman, J.A. (1984) *Biopolymers* 23, 313-323.
[24] Perret, S., Eble, J.A., Siljander, P.R.-M., Merle, C., Farndale, R.W., Theisen, M., and Ruggiero, F. (2003) *J. Biol. Chem.* 278, 29873–29879.

[25] Kunii, S., Morimoto, K., Nagai, K., Sato, K., Saito, T., and Tonomura, B. (2010) *J. Biol. Chem.* 285, 17465–17470.

[26] Morimoto, K., Kunii, S., Hamano, K., and Tonomura, B. (2004) *Biosci. Biotechnol. Biochem.* 68, 861–867.

[27] Privalov, G., Kavina, V., Freire, E., and Privalov, P.L. (1995) *Anal. Biochem.* 232, 79–85.

[28] Nakayama, T., Shirane, J., Hieshima, K., Shibano, M., Watanabe, M., Jin, Z., Nagakubo, D., Saito, T., Shimomura, Y., and Yosie, O. (2006) *Virology* 350, 484–492.

[29] Tiktopulo, E.I., and Kajava, A.V. (1998) *Biochemistry* 37, 8147–8152.

[30] Freudenberg, U., Behrens, S.H., Welzel, P.B., Müller, M., Grimmer, M., Salchert, K., Taeger, T., Schmidt, K., Pompe, W., and Werner, C. (2007) *Biophys. J.* 92, 2108–2119.

In: Type I Collagen
Editor: Gretchen Rivera

ISBN: 978-1-63482-829-1

Chapter 3

Type-I Collagen Characterization of Humans Suffering Osteogenesis Imperfecta: A Skin Study by Second-Harmonic-Generation Microscopy and Texture Analysis

Javier Adur[1,2], Lilia D'Souza-Li[3], Hernandes F. Carvalho[4], Carlos L. Cesar[4] and Víctor H. Casco[1,2]

[1]Microscopy Laboratory Applied to Molecular and Cellular Studies, Bioengineering School; National University of Entre Ríos. Oro Verde, Entre Ríos, Argentina
[2]CITER - Research and Transfer Center of Entre Ríos, Argentina
[3]Center of Investigation in Pediatrics, Faculty of Medical Sciences, University of Campinas, Campinas, S São Paulo, Brazil
[4]INFABiC - National Institute of Science and Technology on Photonics Applied to Cell Biology, Campinas, São Paulo, Brazil

Abstract

Osteogenesis imperfecta (OI) composes a group of inherited connective tissue disorders, mainly characterized by bone fragility. It is primarily caused by mutations in the genes coding for pro-α1 and pro-α2 chains of type I collagen. The primary OI clinical manifestation is related to defective bone type I collagen fibers, although the condition is also displayed in other type I collagen-containing tissues, as skin. This means that the disease signature (collagen fibrils abnormally organized, oddly small, or both) could be readily detected in skin, which is more accessible than bone for ex vivo analysis. The molecular diagnosis of OI is nowadays based on laborious and time-consuming biochemical and/or histological methods, to evaluate the collagen from biopsy-derived dermal fibroblasts. Therefore, there is a clear need to develop a rapid noninvasive method to diagnose OI.

Second Harmonic Generation (SHG) has emerged as a powerful nonlinear optical contrast mechanism with potential to visualize collagen fibers in a variety of connective tissues. SHG signals depend on non-linear interactions of light with a sub-micron noncentrosymmetric environment. Due to the type of fibrillar structure, collagen is one of the major sources of such signals in biological materials. The aim of the present chapter is to show that SHG microscopy, in combination with appropriated quantification methods, applied to human skin provides an OI diagnostic tool to discriminate diseased from normal tissues. Moreover, this method provides a fine tone approach to differentiate clinical sub-types of OI disorders, being highly advantageous over present primarily clinical diagnostic methods, providing fast and clear confirmation.

Introduction

Type I collagen, the most abundant protein component of the skin, tendon and bone extracellular matrixes, is a heterotrimer consisting of two α1(I) and one α2(I) chains encoded by COL1A1 and COL1A2 genes, respectively. Dominant mutations in at least one of the aforementioned genes cause classical *osteogenesis imperfecta* (OI), which is characterized both by susceptibility to fractures from minimal trauma and growth deficiency [1]. OI is classified principally into 4 types based on their clinical and radiological features [2]. After the discovery of COL1A1/2 mutations in all OI types, the four OI types were often used in clinical practice to reflect severity with mild (OI type I), lethal (OI type II), severely deforming (OI type III), and moderately deforming (OI type IV). In 2004, OI types V and VI were added to the former classification [3], and more recently this classification was extended in OI types VII to XII [4]. An important issue to be considered is that, both the prenatal and postnatal OI diagnosis, despite classification, exhibits a continuum of severity. Such clinical characteristics of OI are summarized in Table 1. For prenatal nowadays diagnosis of OI, ultrasonography is the first choice for detecting fetal pathologies [5]. In order to monitor suspected OI type III or type IV, serial ultrasound examinations are required. In the same way, magnetic resonance imaging (MRI) serves as a second-line imaging approach to confirm, correct or complete sonographic data. Because of its high spatial resolution and full imaging of the entire fetus (in all planes regardless of fetal positioning), fetal MRI can be a complementary imaging tool, when prenatal sonography is unable to discriminate between OI and other forms of skeletal dysplasia. In the case of postnatal diagnosis, clinical suspicion (based on recurrent fractures, limbs shortening, bones deformation, short stature, early osteoporosis, blue sclerae, hearing loss, dental problems, and joint laxity) and an skeletal overview (short stature and/or disproportionate stature and/or clinical deformity of long bones) are signs that lead to a preliminary diagnosis [3]. Nevertheless, the confirmation of the disease requires bone biopsy, a highly invasive procedure. The more recent molecular diagnosis of OI are laborious and time consuming methods, consisting of biochemical measurements and/or histological evaluation of the collagen from biopsy-derived dermal fibroblasts [3]. Consequently, there is a growing need to develop a rapid non-invasive method of OI diagnoses. This requirement is especially important during the first months of life, when the diagnosis must be based only on the clinical observation, so it becomes difficult.

In recent years, nonlinear optical (NLO) microscope techniques have experienced an impressive growth in biomedical imaging applied to early diagnosis [6]. NLO methods, coupled with high-resolution microscopy, allow understanding the interactions between cells, extracellular matrix and stroma, in a tissular environment. The main reason to use NLO microscopy is its ability to analyze non-stained live cells and even more important, to perform deep tissue prospection [7].

Table 1. Gene mutations and clinical characteristics of Osteogenesis Imperfecta

Characteristic Type	Gene Mutations	Severity	Congenital Fractures	Bone Deformity	Stature	Hearing Loss
I	COL1A1	mild	no	rarely	normal	60% of cases
II	COL1A1 COL1A2	perinatal lethal	yes	very severe	severely short	not available
III	COL1A1 COL1A2	severe	usually	severe	very short	common
IV	COL1A1 COL1A2	moderate	rarely	mild moderate	variable short	42% of cases
V	absence of COL1A1/2 mutations	moderate	no	moderate	variable	no
VI	absence of COL1A1/2 mutations	moderate	no	moderate	mild short	no
VII	CRTAP	severe to lethal	no	moderate	short	not available
VIII	mutations in LEPRE1	severe to lethal	no	moderate	not available	not available
IX	mutations in PPIB	moderate to lethal	no	moderate/ severe	mild short	not available
X	mutations in SERPINH1	severe	no	moderate/ severe	mild	not available
XI	mutations in FKBP10	mild	no	moderate	mild	not available
XII	mutations in SP7	moderate	rarely	mild	short	not available

One of the most useful NLO techniques for diagnosis applications is the second harmonic generation (SHG) microscopy. SHG is a second order coherent process in which two lower energy photons are up converted to exactly twice the incident frequency (half the wavelength) of an excitation. Biological SHG imaging was first reported in 1986, when Freund investigated the polarity of collagen fibers in rat tail tendon [8]. In 2002, Mohler and Campagnola reported practical implementation of tissue imaging at high resolution and rapid data acquisition, using laser scanning. From that time, SHG microscopy has been increasingly used as imaging tool [9].

Afterward, these authors exploited the sensitivity of SHG to identify supramolecular assemblies and to investigate whether this approach could be used to differentiate normal and OI tissues in a murine model (mOI) with biochemical and phenotypical features similar to those observed in patients with type III OI. The SHG intensity as well as morphological differences allowed them to discriminate the cases [10], especially because mOI matrix was comprised of smaller, more randomly packed fibrils, meaning that these structures have a less organized collagen lattice [10,11]. Recently, in a more inclusive study, our group has showed that SHG microscopy in human skin provides an OI diagnostic, discriminating OI from normal and, moreover, that this method was capable to differentiate the clinical types of OI as well [12]. In that study, we have demonstrated that combining nonlinear microscopy techniques with different scoring methods (collagen density, SHG intensity, ratio between collagen and elastic tissue, and texture analysis) allowed differentiating the classical types of OI advantageously compared to present postnatal diagnostic approaches, which are primarily clinical, without fast and clear confirmatory method.

The present chapter shows how, combining human skin SHG and texture analysis, the accuracy of nonlinear images in the detection of OI may be improved. This chapter first gives an introduction to the relationship between collagen I and OI disease (Section 1). A description of how skin collagen fibers generate nonlinear signal and following, how a SHG microscopy works are summarized in Section 2. The section 3 focuses on both, the different textural parameters definition and also the demonstration of their usefulness to differentiate the morphology and distribution of collagen fibers. Finally, in section 4 it come to highlighting the usefulness of these techniques to differentiate the OI clinical types.

I. Type I Collagen and Osteogenesis Imperfecta

OI is a heterogeneous disorder of connective tissues with an incidence of 1/15000 [13, 14] and disease severity spanning from subclinical osteoporosis to intrauterine lethality. Dominant mutation in collagen type I is the most common cause (> 90%).

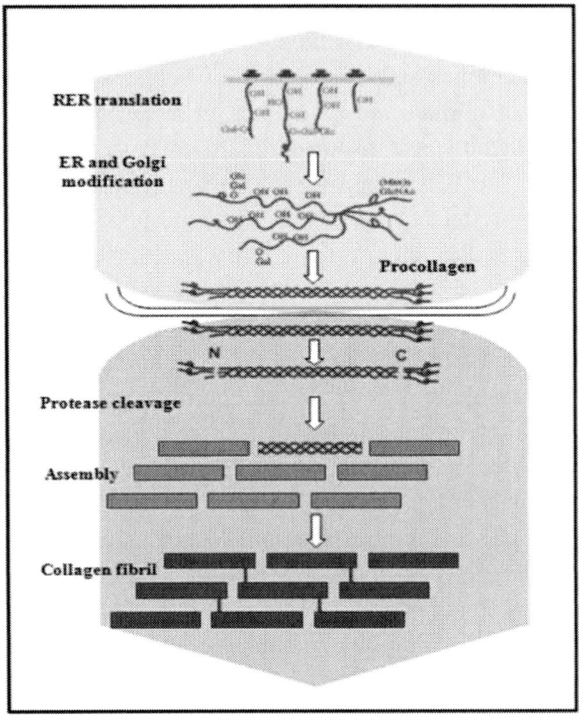

Figure 1. Overview of type I collagen biosynthesis. This fibrous, structural protein consists of a right-handed bundle of three parallel, left-handed polyproline II-type helices, two α1-chains and one α2-chain. After translation, both pro-α1-chains and pro-α2 chains are processed in the rough endoplasmic reticulum (rER). These chains must be aligned in order to start the folding process of (pro)collagen type I into a triple helix. The next step is the alignment of the three chains to initiate the folding in a triple helix structure. During this folding process, post-translational modification by specific proteins takes place. After transport of procollagen type I to the Golgi complex and following exocytosis into the extracellular matrix, cleavage of the C-and N-propeptides results in formation of collagen type I. Subsequently, cross-linking of collagen type I molecules leads to fibrils formation.

Type I collagen is the most abundant extracellular matrix (ECM) protein in humans and the major structural protein in many organs, for example in skin. It is a heterotrimer consisting of two α1-chains and one α2-chain, encoded by COL1A1 and COL1A2 respectively.

The precursor form, type I procollagen, contains a central helical domain, flanked by an amino-(N) and carboxy-(C) terminal pro-peptide. The central helical domain consists of a repeating [Gly-X-Y] triplet in which glycine is the only amino acid small enough to reside within the sterically restricted inner aspect of the helix. Type I procollagen molecules are synthesized and folded in the rough endoplasmic reticulum, where they are modified by hydroxylating and glycosylating enzymes and following are secreted into the ECM. After cleavage of the N- and C-terminal pro-peptide by specific N- and C-proteinases, they are converted to mature collagen molecules, which self-assemble into fibrils (Figure 1).

Mutations in the genes encoding type I procollagen produce a range of disorders, which include autosomal dominant (AD) osteogenesis imperfecta (OI). Currently, more than 1,000 heterozygous COL1A1/2 mutations have been identified (https://oi.gene.le.ac.uk) [15, 16]. Mutation type and position influence the phenotype and as such genotype–phenotype relations exist to some extent. Mainly, two types of mutations in collagen I cause classical dominant OI: quantitative and qualitative collagen defects (Table 1).

Quantitative mutations are the result of haploinsufficiency of COL1A1; patients have structurally normal collagen type I, but the molecule production is significantly reduced. Premature stop codons and splice-site mutations or insertion/deletions are commonly observed mutation types and all cause nonsense-mediated decay of mRNA from one COL1A1 allele. Collagen type I is highly expressed in many connective tissue cell types, and both alleles of COL1A1 are required to meet the organism needs.

Haploinsufficiency of COL1A1 is usually associated with the milder type I phenotype, while COL1A2 haploinsufficiency does not have an overt clinical bone phenotype [17]. Qualitative mutations are generally glycine substitutions (80%) or splice site mutations (20%); however, rare N- and C-terminal and X- and Y-position helical mutations have been described [1, 18-19]. Glycine is the only amino acid small enough to fit in the confined helical center of collagen I, and thus a prerequisite for correct folding. All described helical glycine substitutions cause OI phenotypes, with a severity depending on the position and specific substitution. Qualitative mutations cause a more heterogeneous phenotypic spectrum than quantitative mutations, ranging from mild disease similar to osteoporosis to perinatal lethal OI.

According to previous description, collagen I mutations are reflected in some way on fibril collagen assembly that can be finally observed in an organ, such as skin (Figure 2). For example, in patients suffering OI, skin collagen fibers could be smaller and more randomly packed. These disorders in collagen fibrils could be quantified using SHG microscopy, because this technique has the ability to detect collagen structure alterations.

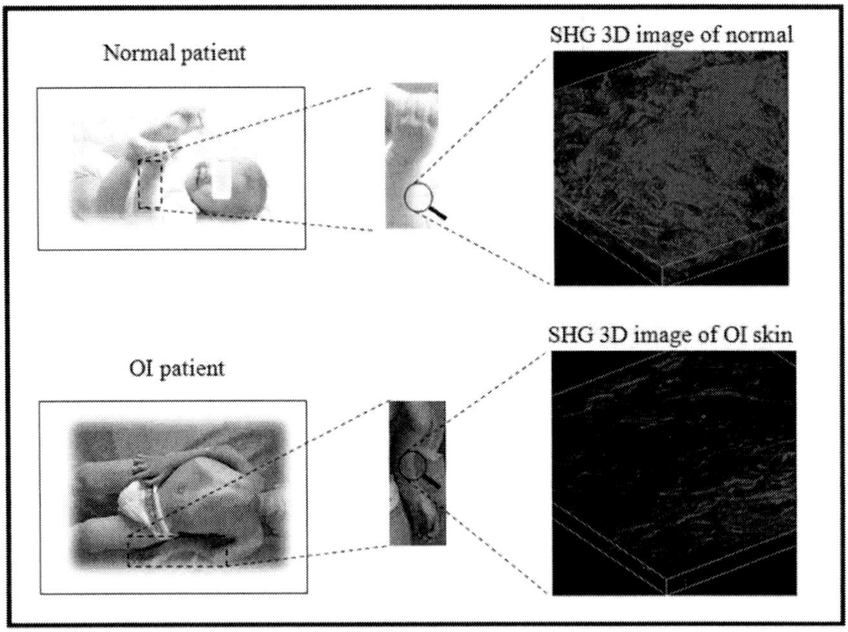

Figure 2. Schematic representation showing how SHG microscopy images from skin could be used to detect collagen structure alterations. Normal individual (upper row) and OI patient (bottom row) with their respective tridimensional representation of SHG images from skin are showed.

SHG signals depend on non-linear interactions light sources with a submicron non-centrosymmetric environment [20, 21]. As was described below, the non-centrosymmetric structure of fibrillar collagen makes it, the major source of the SHG signals in biological materials. Therefore, any modifications in fibrillar collagen should be reflected in changes in SHG signal (Figure 2).

II. SHG Microscopy and Type I Colalagen

II.1. Nonlinear SHG Microscopy

SHG technique is one of the nonlinear optical phenomena that occur when the response of a specimen depends upon the strength of the optical electric field in a nonlinear manner. They occur as a result of that part of the atomic response to the oscillating field of the light that quadratically depends on the strength of this optical field. Consequently, the intensity of the signal generated by the SHG mechanism does increase as the square of the incident light intensity. Since SHG microscopy is based on nonlinear optical processes, it retains the benefits of multi-photon excitation microscopy, such as the intrinsic 3D sectioning ability and relative depth penetration. As different imaging mechanisms from multi-photon absorption, SHG do not involve an excited state (Figure 3), and therefore leave no energy tissular deposition, permitting non-invasive imaging which is desirable for clinical applications.

Furthermore, SHG is a coherent process, where the phase of the radiated harmonic light is tightly matched to the phase of the applied fundamental light, so that harmonic light exhibits a significant dependence on the spatial distributions of both the molecules and the field of the incident fundamental light. This coherence-conserving feature enables the polarization dependence of harmonic light that provides information about molecular organization and nonlinear susceptibility not available from fluorescence light with random phase [22]. SHG is a process where two lower energy photons are up-converted to exactly twice the incident frequency (or half the wavelength) (Figure 3). Another physical implication during the coherent processes is that the harmonic emission is propagated in the forward direction. The second-order susceptibility (χ^2) responsible for SHG only exists in non-centrosymmetric materials [23]. Therefore, SHG shall be zero in the presence of centro-symmetric molecules, unless an external parameter, such as electric fields or interfaces, breaks the symmetry.

SHG imaging mode can probe molecular organization, molecular symmetry, orientation, molecular alignments and ultrastructure at the micro- and nanoscale. Because most biological structures are not highly ordered, they are optically isotropic and do not produce any SHG signal. Only those few biological structures that are ordered or that involve some spatial organizations that break the optical centro-symmetry can produce harmonic signal. Namely collagen, the major protein of the extracellular matrix, is one of the best-known SHG signal generated structures in biology. Collagen fibrils often aggregate into larger, cable-like bundles, several micrometers in diameter. This regularly staggered packing order provides the needed structural conditions for efficient SHG [24] (Figure 3).

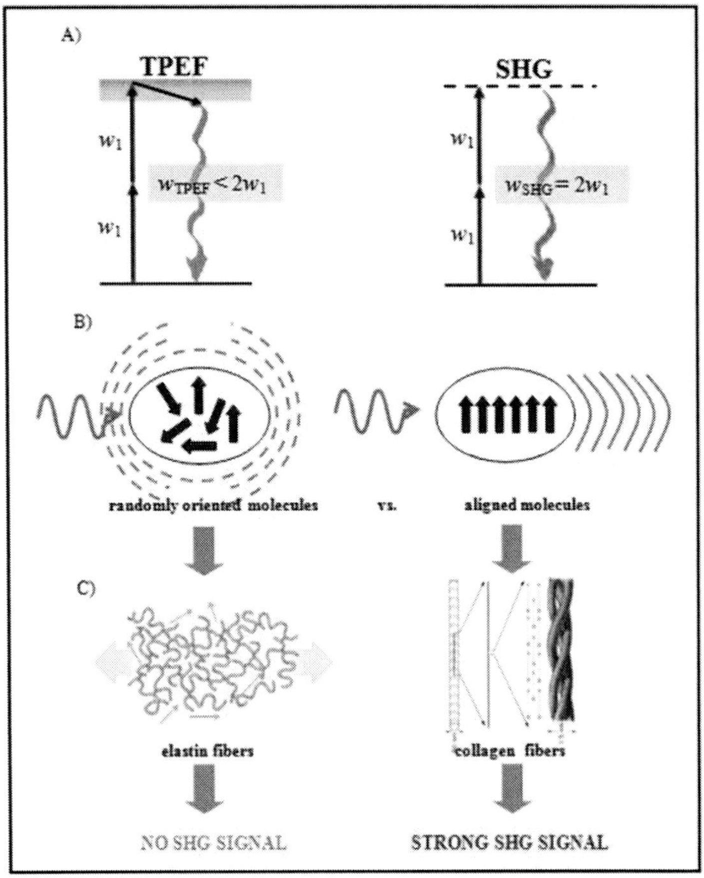

Figure 3. A) Energy diagrams of TPEF (two photon excited fluorescence) and SHG (second harmonic generation) NLO techniques. Solid lines represent electronic and vibrational states of molecules, while dashed lines denote virtual states. The straight arrows are excitation beams, whereas wavy arrows, the output signal beams. ω1 is the frequency from the excitation beams. B) left panel show hyper-Rayleigh incoherent scattering (blue) from a population of N molecules (red) randomly oriented. In right panel, aligned molecules (red) scatter coherently (blue), producing second-harmonic generation (SHG). C) Typical biological examples showing: randomly oriented molecules (elastin - green arrows) that do not generate SHG signal and aligned molecules (collagen - green arrows) producing strong SHG signal.

II.2. SHG Microscopy in Skin

In the past decade, a virtual explosion of research has shown the promise of SHG in tissue imaging. The majority of the recent reports have focused on visualizing collagen fibers in a variety of connective tissues including cornea, skin, tendon, bone, as well as fibrotic collagen in internal organs [25-29]. The efforts over the past decade have established SHG as a viable imaging technique and real-life applications are emerging, especially as a diagnostic tool for diseases and other pathological conditions. Due to the exquisite sensitivity of SHG to supramolecular structure, there is considerable optimism that SHG imaging may be translated to clinical applications. With this aim, we have successfully used SHG, to image and characterize different connective tissue disorders such as in stromal ovary, breast, colon [7, 30-32] (Figure 4). Additionally, others authors were able to search collagen fibers inside skin dermis [33]. SHG was also used for investigating collagen-fiber orientation and their structural changes in fibrotic collagen [34], human dermis [35], and keloid [36]. In healthy dermis, the collagen-fiber bundles are arranged in a parallel way to the epithelial surface, keeping interconnected by fine fibrillar strands of collagen [37]. Cutaneous keloids and hypertrophic scars are examples of abnormal wound healing and are characterized by excessive dermal fibrosis. They are formed during wound healing after skin damage. In a recent work, Cicchi and coworkers using SHG techniques and different image-pattern analysis approaches have showed the capability to characterize skin tissue suffering some particular dermal disorder [38].

LaComb et al., (2008) have demonstrated that, a combined approach of SHG imaging and simulation, can be used to differentiate normal and OI in mouse skin tissues [11]. The overall ensemble of parameters constituting their quantification metric was consistent with a more disordered matrix comprised of smaller fibrils in the OI mouse diseased state. The authors sustain that their results show further consistency between phenotype and genotype and further, that this optical scheme could be used in lieu of current invasive and destructive methods. Based on their finding, they concluded that the approach may be particularly valuable in diagnosing the OI severity and it might allow establish the correlation with the genetic information. Although they do sustained that the diseased signatures would emerge over the inherent tissue heterogeneity, also they estimated that the method would be especially useful in monitoring the status of individual patients relative to their initial screen, where patients would already have a genetic profile [11]. SHG is also well-suited for optical sectioning studies. For example, it is possible, carrying out imaging on *ex vivo* biopsies or ultimately *in vivo*, that the scattering signatures will arise from several layers of the tissue. However, SHG provides isolation of the response from the collagenous layers, corresponding to the dermis. Having the ability to carry out this analysis on skin has the added potential clinical benefit.

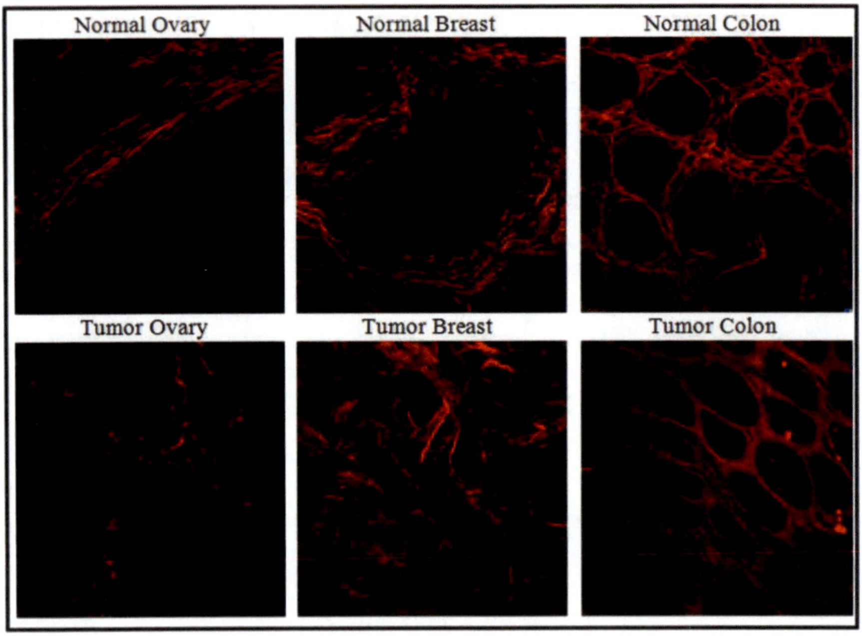

Figure 4. Representative SHG images from different epithelial tissues from normal (upper row) and malignant (bottom row) ovary, breast, and colon respectively. At naked eye it is possible to perceive that collagen fibers become disorganized in pathological tissues.

In order to improve new tools for the diagnosis of this disease based on SHG microscopy, we have recently implemented an optical setup in combination with several quantification methods to demonstrate that quantitative analysis of images from collagen fiber of human skin biopsy could be used to detect OI [12]. A detailed description of such microscopy system is described below.

II.3. SHG Microscopy Setup

The evolution of the SHG microscopy into a viable tool has been enabled by technology developments in suitable off-the-shelf, mode-locked, ultrafast lasers along with the development of laser scanning and data acquisition hardware/software. Figure 5A depicts a diagrammatic representation of a typical imaging system for SHG nonlinear microscope using Ti:Sa lasers. In our setup, the system consisted of an inverted microscope Axio Observer Z.1 equipped with a Zeiss LSM 780-NLO confocal scan head (Carl Zeiss AG, Germany). The excitation beam was provided by a mode-locked Ti:Sapphire laser (Spectra-Physics. Irvine, USA) emitting at 100-fs width pulses, 80 MHz repetition rate, 940 nm of wavelength and an average power at the sample of 10 mW.

This laser system was equipped with a DeepSee for group velocity dispersion compensation and an acousto-optic modulator (AOM) for laser power attenuation. The beam was coupled to the scan head after a collimating telescope (T1). We used circular polarized light to avoid anisotropies for different fibril's directions. To do that, we placed a broadband quarter waveplate (l/4-Newport) in the laser beam before the microscope scan head and rotating this plate until the light power after the objective did not change with a rotation of a polarizer.

The beam was focused onto the sample by a 40X/ 1.30 NA oil immersion objective (EC Plan-Neofluar Carl Zeiss AG, Germany). The forward propagating SHG (470 nm) and two-photon fluorescence signals (>490 nm) were collected by the condenser lens 0.55 NA – WD 26 mm (Carl Zeiss) and acquired simultaneously by non-descanned detector (NDD) after a blocking filter SP720 (Omega Filters) to prevent back-reflected laser light.

A filter cube with a dichroic LP490 nm wavelength (Carl Zeiss part number 1481-247) and a filter SP485 nm wavelength (Carl Zeiss part number 1481-370) were placed ahead the SHG detector to cut out unwanted fluorescence light from the SHG channel. Other filter cube with a mirror (Carl Zeiss part number 1512-461) and a narrow (20 nm FWHM) BP540 filter (Carl Zeiss part number 1443-332) was used to detect TPEF signal.

Figure 5B shows representative images acquired by using this configuration, displaying representative TPEF and SHG images (with 512x512 pixel spatial resolution). TPEF is generated fundamentally by the eosin fluorescence and, in every case this signal was used, to detect just the skin epithelium (dashed white line). The non-contamination confirmation of the SHG signal was established by the wavelength range, half of the excitation, of the signal, by using the Avalanche Photodiodes (APD) array of the LSM-780 Zeiss scan head CCD.

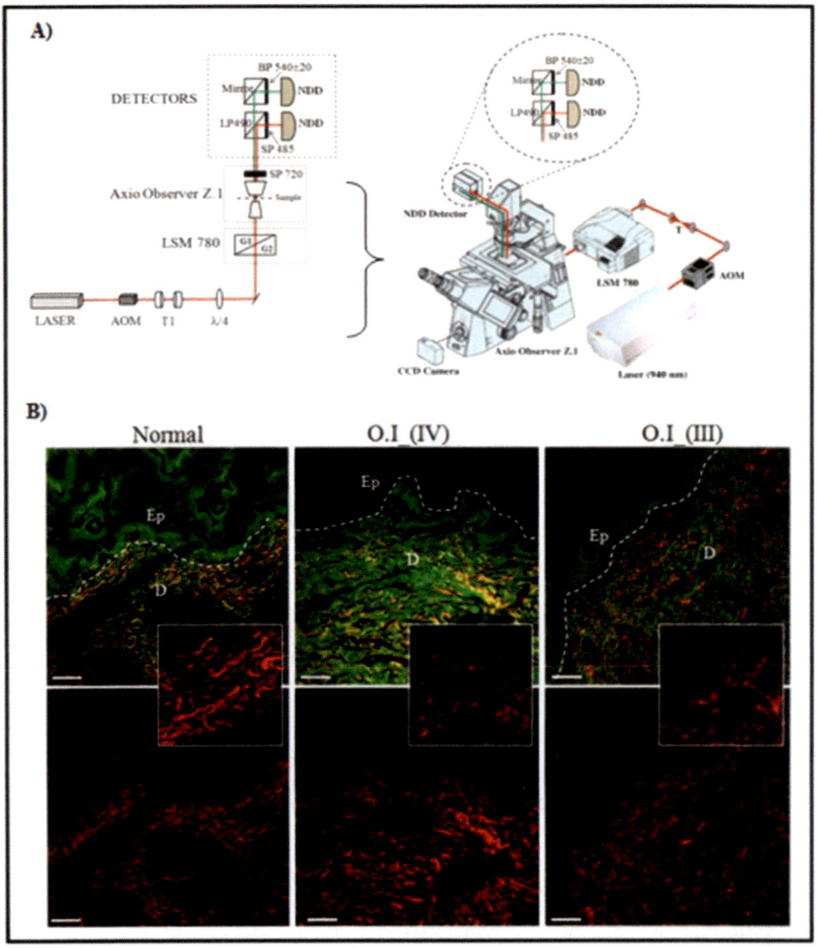

Figure 5. A) Experimental setup to TPEF and SHG microscopy based on an inverted microscope Axio Observer Z.1 and LSM 780-NLO confocal scan head (Carl Zeiss AG, Germany), AOM: acoust-optic modulator, T1: telescope, l/4: quarter waveplate, G1/G2: galvanometer mirrors, SP: short-pass filter, BP: bandpass filter, LP: long-pass filter, NDD: Non Descanned Detector. The SHG (red lines) and TPEF (green lines) are collected in a transmitted light configuration. B) Representative cross-sectional images obtained with setup show in A) for TPEF and SHG analyses of normal, OI type IV, and OI type III skin human tissues. Epidermis/dermis interface is signposted by white outline. Insets highlight visual differences of fiber collagen. Ep: epidermis; and D: dermis.

These skin images are just a basic representative example about how the SHG tool can be used in future in vivo optical evaluation of OI. However, we are aware that it is necessary to develop reliable quantitative methods to discriminate between different types of OI. This requirement is really important if this tool is to be used for clinical diagnostic purposes. The following section has the main objective to demonstrate that the texture analyses will be a first step to provide a SHG images quantitation tool, providing important information about collagen fibers organization.

III. Texture Analysis

In order to accomplish potential efficient, accurate and objective clinical diagnoses methods, the morphology of collagen fibers revealed by SHG imaging has been quantitatively described by texture analysis. Texture analysis approaches can be categorized into statistical, structural, model-based, and transform-based methods [39]. For medical applications, the statistical methods are extensively used, since they can provide higher discrimination indexes [40]. As the most frequently cited statistical method [39, 40], the gray level co-occurrence matrix (GLCM) has been applied to a variety of fields for decades, including texture analysis of medical images [41, 42]. Combined with SHG imaging, the GLCM approach has been applied to quantitatively analyze the collagen fibers [38].

The GLCM analysis method allows the classification of different tissues based on the evaluation of geometrical collagen arrangement. It provides information on the spatial relationships between pixel brightness values in a given image. The GLCM is constructed by counting the number of occurrences of a gray level adjacent to another gray level, at a specified pixel distance "*d*" and dividing each counting by the total counting number to obtain a probability. The result is a matrix with rows and columns representing gray levels and elements containing the probability P_d [i,j] of the gray level co-occurrence between pixels. The matrix is usually averaged in opposite and different orientations (0–180°, 45–225°, 90–270°, and 135–315°) unless the one-dimensional feature dominates over all possible ones, in which case, the 0–180° average is sufficient. A detailed explanation on how this matrix is created from the original image can be reviewed in [38, 43].

The GLCM analysis can be carried out by different methods; they are commonly classified as contrast, orderliness and statistical methods. Contrast methods can be employed in order to give quantitative information on the intensity fluctuations in the image. Among the contrast methods, homogeneity is the weighted sum of the GLCM pixel values. The weights are values that decrease nonlinearly as the distance from the GLCM matrix diagonal increases. Homogeneity gives information on the similarity of a pixel value in combination with its neighboring pixel to all the other pairs of neighboring pixels in the image.

Orderliness methods are particularly applicable to images containing fibrillar structures such as SHG images of collagen, and they can be employed in order to give a quantitative measurement on the mutual orientation of collagen fiber bundles.

Table 2. GLCM parameters and its mathematical expressions

Parameters	Interpretation	Mathematical Expression
Correlation	Linear dependency of grey levels on those of neighboring pixels	$-\sum_{i,j=0}^{N-1} P_{i,j}\left[\frac{(i-\mu)(j-\mu)}{\sigma^2}\right]$
Contrast	Representation of pixels entirely similar to their neighbor	$\sum_{i,j=0}^{N-1} (i-j)^2 P_{i,j}$
Energy	Degree of image´s texture directions according to the perception of human eyes	$\sum_{i,j=0}^{N-1} P_{i,j}^2$
Homogeneity	Measure of the amount of local uniformity present in the image	$\sum_{i,j=0}^{N-1} \frac{P^2{}_{i,j}}{1+(i-j)^2}$

GLCM: gray level co-occurrence matrix; *P*: probability density function; *i-j*: gray levels.

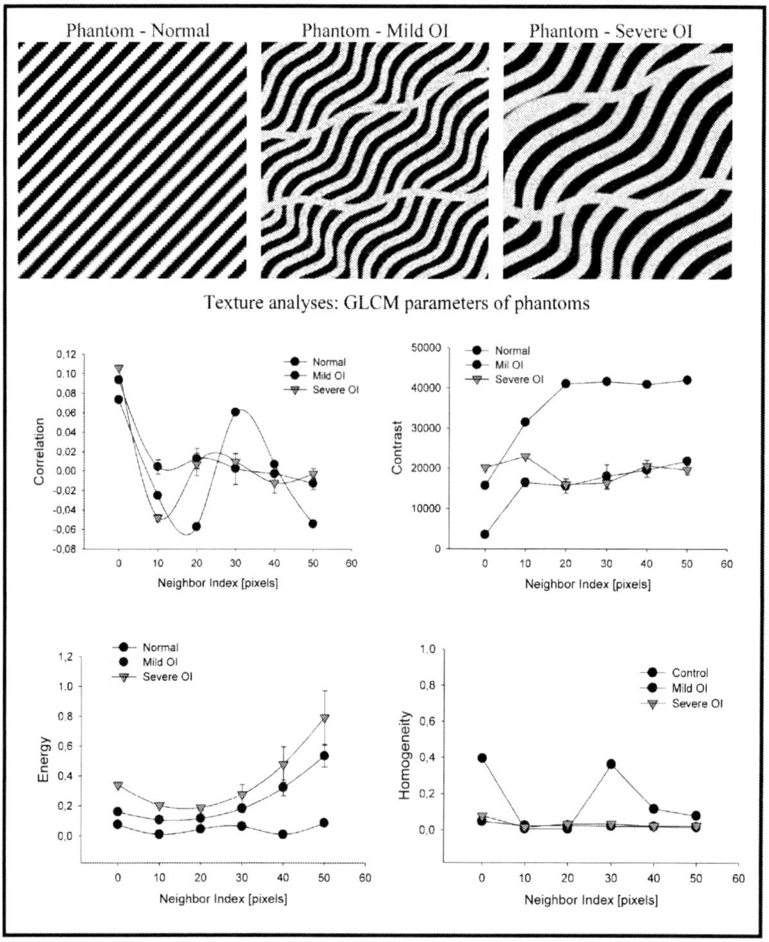

Figure 6. GLCM analysis was performed in phantom images consisting of strips arranged in regular (normal and mild OI) and random structure (severe OI). The strips widths are manually establish in 13 pixels for normal collagen fibers and 20 pixels for severe OI representation. Each curve shows different GLCM parameter calculated for normal (black), mild OI (red), and severe OI (green). For calculations, non symmetric GLCMs were computed using 256 gray-levels. For a 354.3 μm x 354.3μm (1024x1024 pixels) image, a practical upper bound on pixel separation is 50 pixels. Separations of 1 to 50 in 1-pixel increments were used for this study. The aim of the next section is to show that SHG microscopy is capable to differentiate the clinical types of OI, when is combined with texture analysis quantification.

For example, energy is the root squared sum of the GLCM pixel values. Considering that this parameter gives higher weight to the hot spots of the GLCM matrix, energy is a measure of orderliness of the image. Finally, statistical methods are based on the statistical analysis of pixel value dependence, and they can be used for determining repetition of a certain pattern within an image. Among them, the correlation method probably represents the most powerful approach to be applied to SHG images of collagen.

The parameters used in this chapter, their significance and mathematical expression are shown in table 2. For $d = 0$, then $i = j$, and therefore correlation and homogeneity take the value 1, and energy is any number between 0 and 1. The texture analyses can be performed with ImageJ GLCM Texture plugin, which was described by Walker and coworkers [44].

To validate the dependence of GLCM analysis of collagen fibers, we have built phantom images with different orientations, which consist of strips with regular separation (simulating normal skin) and structure with random separation and thicker strips (simulating skin with OI) (figure 6). The white strips were manually created by and converted to gray-level synthetic images with 512×512 pixels. The width of the strips are manually set to be 13 pixels according previous morphology definitions for normal collagen fibers [12,45] and 20 pixels for severe OI representation.

According to figure 6, the images with a relatively regular texture and thin strips (normal and mild OI phantom) shows lower energy and higher contrast (normal phantom). Normal phantom representing healthy collagen is more ordered (thin strip produce more quickly pixels variations), what is evidenced by the high contrast levels, compared with pathological ones. Since strips width and spacing affects the gray levels transition across the image, it is expected that GLCM energy will change for different strips morphologies. Well oriented fibers have lower average energy because they are thinner, causing more variation in gray levels when moving across the image. Latter we shall see that this is the parameter with better performance to differentiate abnormal collagen fibers.

IV. SHG Microscopy and Texture Analysis for OI

Skin samples from healthy and from patients with OI came from the Laboratory of Pediatric Endocrinology, Campinas, SP, Brazil. All procedures were approved by the local Research Institutional Ethics Committee and in accordance with the Declaration of Helsinki and the ethical principles of the medical community. Biopsies were analyzed and classified as normal (4 cases) or OI (5 cases). OI patients were classified according to clinical observations in mild OI (Type I - 1 case), moderately affected and severe OI (Type III or Type IV - 4 cases). Table 3 shows clinical characteristics of these patients and molecular analysis with mutations found in COL1A1 or COL1A2 genes confirming the qualitative defects in collagen type I. Normal samples were obtained from eyelid plastic surgery discarded tissue and patient`s biopsy were obtained from growing skin. Fresh skin samples in PBS solution were analyzed by 3D SHG representations within 6 hs of the excision. From the mounted SHG pictures, we took images located in the dermis. Non symmetric GLCMs were computed using 256 gray-levels. Because collagen fiber orientation changed from sample to sample, four orientations average were used.

Table 3. Patients characteristic

Patient	OI Type	Age	Severity	Fractures	Bone Def.	Stature	Gen
A	I	20	mild	infrequent	absent	normal	*COL1A2*
B	IV	42	moderate	infrequent	moderate	short	*COL1A1*
C	IV	12	moderate	infrequent	moderate	short	*COL1A1*
D	IV	21	severe	frequent	moderate	short	*COL1A1* *COL1A2*
E	III	21	severe	frequent	severe	short	*COL1A2*

Starting from a superficial inspection of the SHG images (Figure 7) can be clearly visualized that the normal skin had thinner collagen fibers that weaved in all directions around the hair follicles. The skin from OI patients presented more variation in collagen fiber thickness when compared to the normal ones. Skin images from the more severe forms of OI (type III and IV) tended to have thicker, broken and wavy collagen fibers that were packed together in the same direction.

The quantitation of these qualitative approaches was done using the texture parameters depicted in figure 8, from representative images. Specifically, correlation (Figure 8B), contrast (Figure 8C), energy (Figure 8D), and homogeneity (Figure 8E) values were obtained for analyzes purposes. More severe OI forms (type III and IV) are greatest differentiated from normal and from mild OI (type I) by three GLCM parameters: contrast, energy, and homogeneity. Homogeneity and energy gave similar results because they are not completely independent of each other, even if they are correlated to contrast and orderliness of the image, respectively. Among the four curves extracted from texture analysis, the energy and contrast at different pixel separations are the most sensitive, showing a statistically significant differences ($p< 0.05$) when normal skin is compared with OI patient´s skin. Since collagen fiber width and spacing affects the gray levels transition across the image, it is expected that GLCM energy will change for different collagen morphologies. Normal fibers have lower average energy because they are thinner, causing more variation in gray levels when moving across the image.

A more complete quantification using energy-GLCM parameter is shown in figure 9.

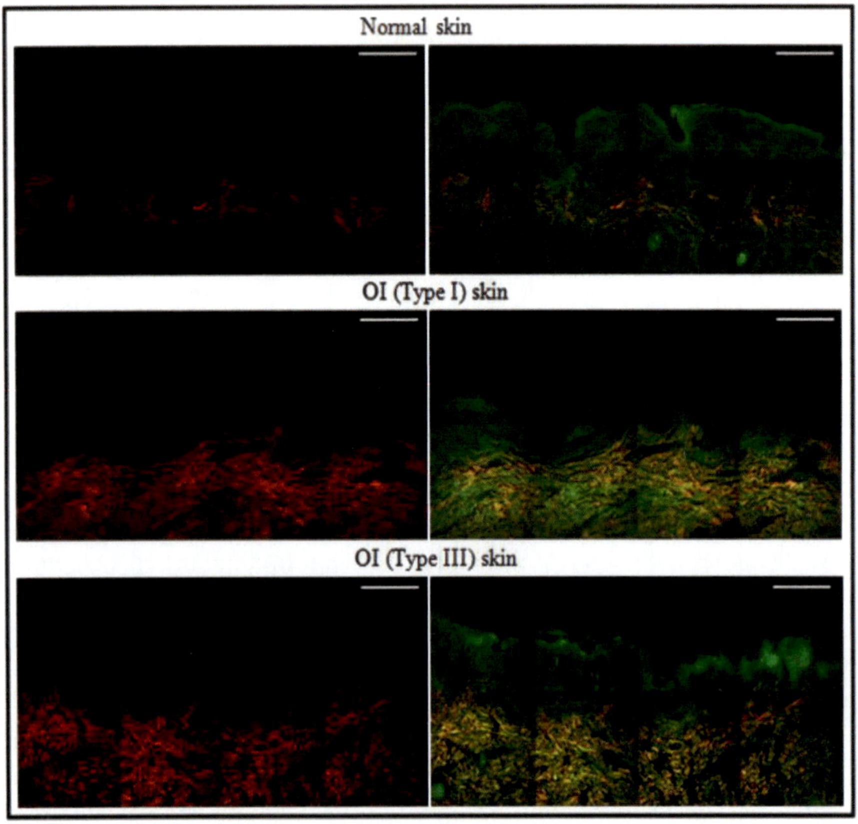

Figure 7. Montage of SHG red and TPEF+SHG green and red images. Representative images of fixed normal skin from control, Type I OI patient and Type III OI patients. Scale bar = 200 μm.

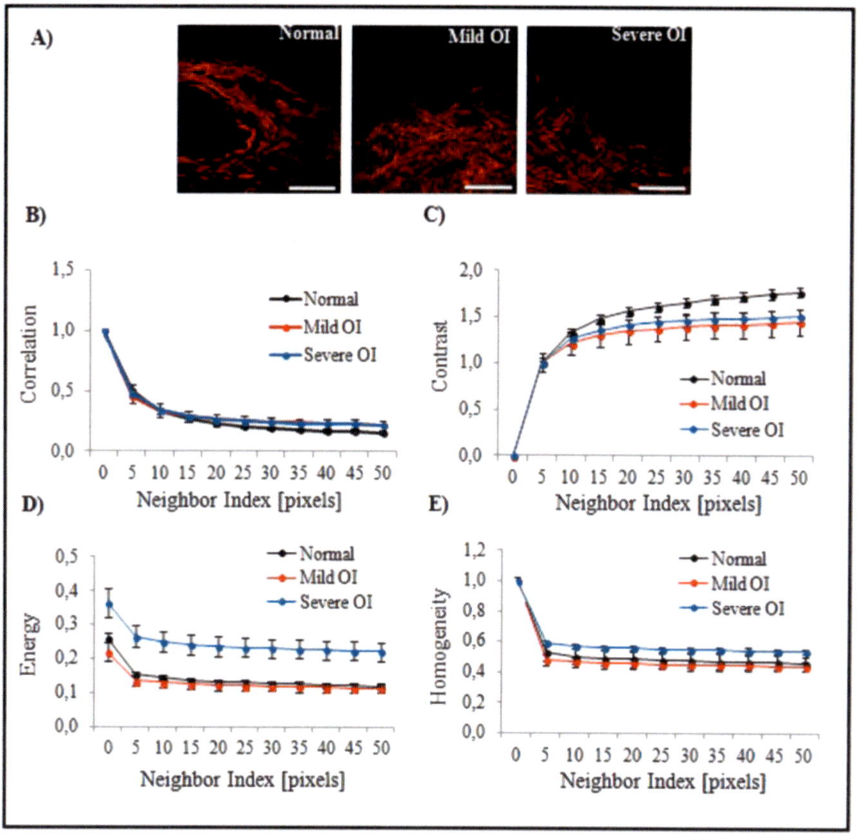

Figure 8. Texture analysis of skin dermis. A) One representative SHG image (354.30 x 354.30 μm) of the eight images from figure 7. Normal skin (first column), OI-Type I (second column), and OI-Type III (third column). Scale bars = 100 μm. Texture analysis using the gray-level co-occurrence matrix (GLCM). Correlation (B), Contrast (C), Energy (D), and Homogeneity (E) values in dermis tissues versus distance pixels; ranging from 1 to 50 pixels (0.35μm–17.30μm) in 0, 45, 90 and 135 deg directions of image. (n = 12 normal, n = 3 mild OI, and n = 9 severe OI). Black line (normal), red line (mild OI), and blue line (severe OI).

This scoring method was competent to satisfactorily discriminate the different OI patients according to their clinical severity. Using fresh biopsies, one could detect a marked density decrease of the collagen fibers network in the 3D representations of SHG images from severe OI patient's samples (Figure 9B (Type III) and Figure 9C (Type IV)), when compared with the 3D representation of SHG images taken from normal skin fresh biopsies (Figure 9A). Furthermore, energy value of GLCM texture analysis not only able to discriminate type I and type III OI samples, from normal skin (Figure 9D) but it could also differentiate (with statistical significance) between patients with varying degrees of OI, including type IV OI (Figure 9E).

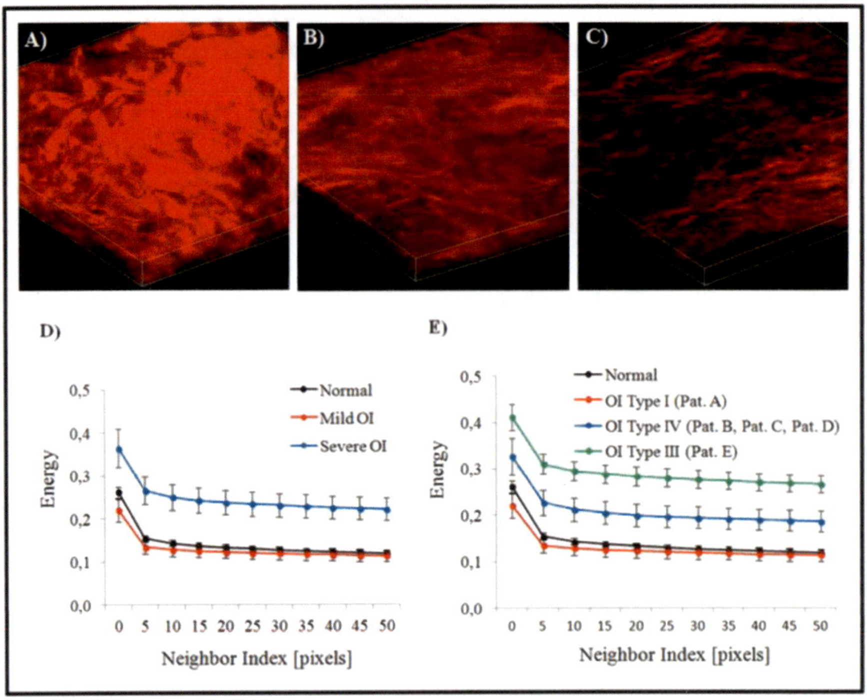

Figure 9. Representative 3D maximum projection (40 images at 1 μm intervals) of SHG images from fresh skin biopsies, A: normal skin, B: OI Type III (Patient E) and C: OI Type IV (Patient D). Texture analysis (D, E), using the gray-level co-occurrence matrix (GLCM). Energy values were calculated in dermis tissues versus distances pixels; ranging from 1 to 50 pixels (0.35 μm - 17.30 μm) in 0, 45, 90 and 135 deg directions of image (D: n = 12 normal, n = 3 mild OI, and n = 12 severe OI; and E: n = 12 normal, n = 3 OI Type I, n = 9 OI Type IV, n = 3 OI Type III). Pat: patients.

It is very well known that dermis collagen fibers have diameter ranges around 0.5 to 3 μm. Therefore, it is expected that GLCM analysis would show a repeating structure with distances of about 1.5–8 pixels correspondingly to the 0.5–3 μm range. Considering that OI patients exhibit thicker fibers than normal skin samples, GLCM correlation signals could be to drop on a longer scale. The values of decay length are obtained by fitting the correlation data with a double exponential decay function (red curve, Figure 10).

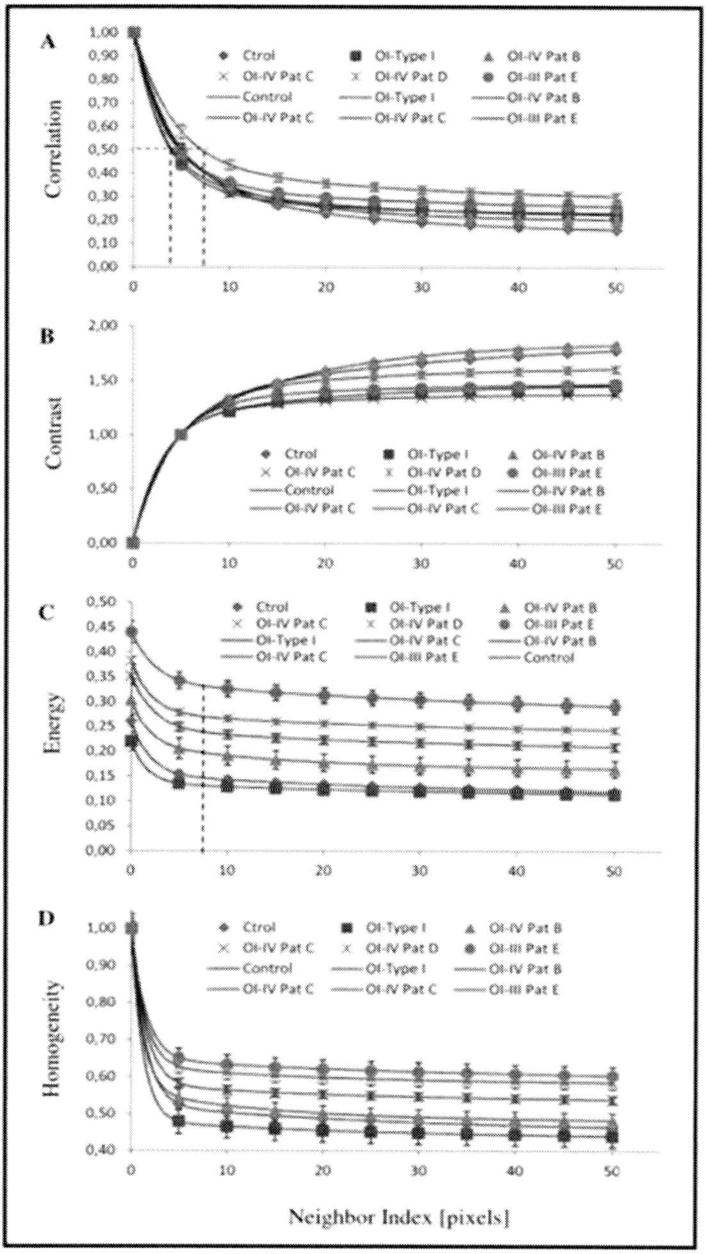

Figure 10. Texture analysis using the gray-level co-occurrence matrix (GLCM). The plots were fit (red curve) with a constant background of two exponentials using the following formula: $y = a0 + a1.e^{(-1x/x1)} + a2.e^{(-1x/x2)}$. Correlation (A), Contrast (B),

Energy (C), and Homogeneity (D) values in dermis tissues versus distances pixels; ranging from 1 to 50 pixels (0.35μm - 17.30μm) in 0, 45, 90 and 135 deg directions of image. (n = 12 normal, n = 3 OI Type I Patient A, n = 3 OI Type IV Patient B, n = 3 OI Type IV Patient C, n = 3 OI Type IV Patient D, and n = 3 OI Type III Patient E). Pat: patients.

The decay length values using the $Corr_{50}$ (the pixel distance where the correlation dropped below 50% of the initial value) obtained are among 1.3 to 2.5 μm (3.8 - 7 pixels) (Figure 10A) confirming that patient D had thicker collagen fiber ≈ 2.5 μm (7 pixels). Using this pixel distance as comparison, the Energy parameter shows values of 0.15±0.02 (Normal), 0.13±0.04 (Pat. A), 0.20±0.03 (Pat. B), 0.24±0.04 (Pat. C), 0.29±0.03 (Pat. D), and 0.33±0.04 (Pat. E), with significant differences ($p<0.05$) when normal skin was compared with OI patient´s (B, C, D and E) skin. This means that this texture parameter clearly allows the identification of each patient pattern (Figure 10C). Interestingly, one of type IV patient exhibiting a more severe phenotype (Patient D) than the others, with a degree of bone fragility that limited her mobility and confined her to a wheelchair. SHG images of these patients skin show a more compacted collagen pattern (thicker collagen fiber), intermediate between type III and the two remaining type IV patients.

This preliminary results, allow to augur that these nonlinear microscopy techniques in association with specific scoring method (energy-GLCM) will be an excellent diagnostic tool to clinically distinguish different types of OI in human skin. This approach may be particularly valuable in diagnosing the severity of OI allowing their correlation with genetic information. We propose that this method could be an excellent complement of the current clinical diagnosis tools (see Table 4) and may be used either as a diagnostic tool or as way to measure of treatment efficacy.

Table 4. SHG diagnosis of OI

OI Type	Severity	Congenital fractures	Bone deformation	SHG + GLCM (energy value d = 7)
Normal				Low (0.15)
I	mild	no	rarely	Low (0.13)
II	severe lethal	yes	very severe	Not available
III	severe	yes	moderate severe	High (0.33)
IV	moderate	rarely	mild severe	Medium (0.24)

Conclusion

The results on the OI human skin show that energy-GLCM pattern provides a quantitative method to differentiate healthy and diseased tissues. First, we have demonstrated that SHG provides higher-resolution and higher-contrast visualizations of the collagen assembly than the classical observation of histological stained samples. Additionally, classical histological procedures by pathologist have limitations to visualize collagen structural variation into the depth tissue sections for which a 3D reconstruction, based on serial sections, is much more complicate than a 3D reconstruction based on deep nonlinear confocal microscopy. Secondly, the correlation plots show that decay curve were similar in all samples analyzed, revealing that collagen fibers are organized similarly and with certain periodicity. However, using texture analysis, we have demonstrated that, even if both mild and severe OI exhibit fibrillar collagen similarly organized in fibers and bundles, the dimension of individual fibers differed between OI types. Also statistically significant differences in contrast (Figure 8C) and energy values (Figure 8D) are observed. Normal skin images show higher contrast values because have high number of pixel pairs with large differences in gray levels occurring at the specified separation and orientation, while the OI skin images present more pixels with similar gray levels. These similarities in gray levels were confirmed by energy and homogeneity values (Figure 8D and E). Severe OI exhibits higher energy (low variation in gray levels) regarding to normal and mild OI (high variation in gray levels). Therefore, this approach allows us to use quantitative comparisons of the structural organization based on differences of the collagen fiber width and spacing. More compact collagen fibers results in higher energy values.

To date, OI diagnosis is based on clinical follow up of radiological and densitometric evaluations, methods that not always allow discriminating the clinical variability within the same OI type. The diagnosis classification does not take these differences into consideration. In this way, despite the small number of patients, we were able to demonstrate that these optical techniques can be used not only to discriminate mild or severe OI from normal skin but also to prove a principle of a diagnostic method to differentiate from an collagen signature (with statistical significance) the different types and clinical severities of OI.

SHG microscopy images of collagen do not require biopsy tissue, neither fixation, sectioning, or staining methods, increasing -considering quantitative approach- its potential use as a diagnostic, besides its valuable use as a research tool. This also means that samples can be preserved for normal procedure diagnostics. In this chapter, we demonstrated the usefulness of SHG microscopy to quantify transformations in human skin dermis of patients suffering OI. Although the most dramatic clinical presentation of OI are present in bone tissues, skin was selected by its accessibility and considering that the goal is to develop SHG imaging as a non-invasive clinical diagnostic tool.

This procedure could be used in lieu of existing invasive, time consuming and destructive methods (such as biochemical measurements, histologic or biochemical evaluation of the collagen from biopsy-derived dermal fibroblasts, and also from bone biopsies), and may be especially useful in monitoring the status of individual patients relative to their initial screen, where patients would already have a genetic profile. Since at present, there is no fast and clear method to diagnose OI, the SHG imaging plus texture analysis can be a very practical method to define the diagnosis, especially with improvements and automatic quantification procedures.

References

[1] Marini JC, Forlino A, Cabral WA, Barnes AM, San Antonio JD, et al. (2007) Consortium for osteogenesis imperfecta mutations in the helical domain of type I collagen: regions rich in lethal mutations align with collagen binding sites for integrins and proteoglycans. *Hum. Mutat.* 28: 209–221.

[2] Sillence DO, Senn A, Danks DM (1979) Genetic heterogeneity in osteogenesis imperfecta. *J. Med. Genet.* 16: 101–116.

[3] van Dijk FS, Cobben JM, Kariminejad A, Maugeri A, Nikkels PGJ, et al. (2011) Osteogenesis Imperfecta: A Review with Clinical Examples. *Mol. Syndromol.* 2:1–20.

[4] Lindahl K, Langdahl B, Ljunggren Ö, Kindmark A. (2014) Treatment of osteogenesis imperfecta in adults. *Eur. J. Endocrinol.* 171(2):R79-R90.

[5] Feng ZY1, Chen Q, Shi CY, Wen HW, Ma K, Yang HX. (2012) A type IV osteogenesis imperfecta family and pregnancy: a case report and literature review. *Chin. Med. J.* 125(7):1358-1360.

[6] Campagnola P. (2011). Second harmonic generation imaging microscopy: applications to diseases diagnostics. *Anal. Chem.* 83(9):3224-3231. Review.

[7] Adur J, Pelegati VB, de Thomaz AA, D'Souza-Li L, Assunção Mdo C, Bottcher-Luiz F, Andrade LA, Cesar CL. (2012) Quantitative changes in human epithelial cancers and osteogenesis imperfecta disease detected using nonlinear microscopy. *J. Biomed. Opt.* 17(8):081407-1.

[8] Freund I, Deutsch M, Sprecher A. (1986) Connective tissue polarity. Optical second-harmonic microscopy, crossed-beam summation, and small-angle scattering in rat-tail tendon. *Biophys. J.* 50(4):693-712.

[9] Campagnola PJ, Millard AC, Terasaki M, Hoppe PE, Malone CJ, Mohler WA. (2012) Three-dimensional high-resolution second-harmonic generation imaging of endogenous structural proteins in biological tissues. *Biophys. J.* 82(1):493-508.

[10] Nadiarnykh O, Plotnikov S, Mohler WA, Kalajzic I, Redford-Badwal D, Campagnola PJ. (2007) Second harmonic generation imaging microscopy studies of osteogenesis imperfecta. *J. Biomed. Opt.* 12(5):051805.

[11] Lacomb R, Nadiarnykh O, Campagnola PJ. (2008) Quantitative second harmonic generation imaging of the diseased state osteogenesis imperfecta: experiment and simulation. *Biophys. J.* 94(11):4504-4514.

[12] Adur J, DSouza-Li L, Pedroni MV, Steiner CE, Pelegati VB, de Thomaz AA, Carvalho HF, Cesar CL. (2013) The severity of Osteogenesis imperfecta and type I collagen pattern in human skin as determined by nonlinear microscopy: proof of principle of a diagnostic method. *PLoS One.* 8(7):e69186.

[13] Kuurila K, Kaitila I, Johansson R, Grenman R. (2002) Hearing loss in Finnish adults with osteogenesis imperfecta: a nation wide survey. *Annals of Otology, Rhinology, and Laryngology* 111: 939–1946.

[14] Stoll C, Dott B, Roth MP, Alembik Y. (1989) Birth prevalence rates of skeletal dysplasias. *Clinical Genetics* 35:88–92.

[15] Dalgleish R. (1997) The human type I collagen mutation database. *Nucleic Acids Res.* 25:181-187.

[16] Dalgleish R. (1998) The human collagen mutation database 1998. *Nucleic Acids Res.* 26:253-255.

[17] Schwarze U, Hata R, McKusick VA, Shinkai H, Hoyme HE, Pyeritz RE, Byers PH. (2004) Rare autosomal recessive cardiac valvular form of Ehlers–Danlos syndrome results from mutations in the COL1A2 gene that activate the nonsense-mediated RNA decay pathway. *American Journal of Human Genetics* 74:917–930.

[18] Cabral WA, Makareeva E, Letocha AD, Scribanu N, Fertala A, Steplewski A, Keene DR, Persikov AV, Leikin S, Marini JC. (2007) Y-

position cysteine substitution in type I collagen (a1(I) R888C/p.R1066C) is associated with osteogenesis imperfecta/Ehlers-Danlos syndrome phenotype. *Human Mutation* 28:396-405.

[19] Pace JM, Wiese M, Drenguis AS, Kuznetsova N, Leikin S, Schwarze U, Chen D, Mooney SH, Unger S, Byers PH. Defective C-propeptides of the proalpha2(I) chain of type I procollagen impede molecular assembly and result in osteogenesis imperfecta. *Journal of Biological Chemistry* 283:16061-16067.

[20] Provenzano PP, Eliceiri KW, Yan L, Ada-Nguema A, Conklin MW, et al. (2008) Nonlinear optical imaging of cellular processes in breast cancer. *Microsc. Microanal.* 14: 532–548.

[21] Cox G, Kable E, Jones A, Fraser I, Manconi F, et al. (2003) 3-dimensional imaging of collagen using second harmonic generation. *J. Struct. Biol* 141: 53–62.

[22] P Stoller, K M Reiser, P M Celliers, A M Rubenchik. (2002) Polarization-modulated second harmonic generation in collagen. *Biophys. J.* 82:3330-3342.

[23] Y R Shen. (1984) The Principles of Nonlinear Optics. New York, John Wiley.

[24] Williams RM, Zipfel WR, Webb WW. Interpreting second-harmonic generation images of collagen I fibrils. *Biophys. J.* 2005; 88:1377-1386.

[25] Yeh AT, Nassif N, Zoumi A, Tromberg BJ. (2002) Selective corneal imaging using combined second-harmonic generation and two-photon excited fluorescence. *Opt. Lett.* 27(23):2082-2084.

[26] Tai SP, Tsai TH, Lee WJ, Shieh DB, Liao YH, Huang HY, Zhang K, Liu HL, Sun CK. (2005) Optical biopsy of fixed human skin with backward-collected optical harmonics signals. *Opt. Express.* 13(20):8231-8242.

[27] Theodossiou TA, Thrasivoulou C, Ekwobi C, Becker DL. (2006) Second harmonic generation confocal microscopy of collagen type I from rat tendon cryosections. *Biophys. J.* 91(12):4665-4677.

[28] Ambekar R, Chittenden M, Jasiuk I, Toussaint KC Jr. (2012) Quantitative second-harmonic generation microscopy for imaging porcine cortical bone: comparison to SEM and its potential to investigate age-related changes. *Bone.* 50(3):643-650.

[29] Strupler M, Pena AM, Hernest M, Tharaux PL, Martin JL, Beaurepaire E, Schanne-Klein MC. (2007) Second harmonic imaging and scoring of collagen in fibrotic tissues. *Opt. Express.* 15(7):4054-4065.

[30] Adur J, Pelegati VB, de Thomaz AA, Baratti MO, Almeida DB, Andrade LA, Bottcher-Luiz F, Carvalho HF, Cesar CL. (2012) Optical biomarkers of serous and mucinous human ovarian tumor assessed with nonlinear optics microscopies. *PLoS One* 7(10):e47007.

[31] Adur J, Pelegati VB, de Thomaz AA, Baratti MO, Andrade LA, Carvalho HF, Bottcher-Luiz F, Cesar CL. (2014) Second harmonic generation microscopy as a powerful diagnostic imaging modality for human ovarian cancer. *J. Biophotonics*. 7(1-2):37-48.

[32] Bianchi M, Adur J, Ruff SY, Izaguirre MF, Carvalho HF, Cesar CL, Casco VH. (2014) Mouse colorectal cancer an early detection approach using nonlinear microscopy. *Biomed. Mater. Eng*. 24(6):3419-3426.

[33] Zipfel WR, Williams RM, Christie R, Nikitin AY, Hyman BT, Webb WW. (2003) Live tissue intrinsic emission microscopy using multiphoton-excited native fluorescence and second harmonic generation. *Proc. Natl. Acad. Sci. U S A*. 100(12):7075-7080.

[34] M Strupler, A M Pena, M Hernest, P L Tharaux, J L Martin, E Beaurepaire, M C Schanne-Klein (2007) Second harmonic imaging and scoring of collagen in fibrotic tissues, *Opt. Exp*. 15, 4054-4065.

[35] Su PJ, Chen WL, Hong JB, Li TH, Wu RJ, Chou CK, Chen SJ, Hu C, Lin SJ, Dong CY. (2009) Discrimination of collagen in normal and pathological skin dermis through second-order susceptibility microscopy. *Opt. Express* 17(13):11161-11171.

[36] Da Costa V1, Wei R, Lim R, Sun CH, Brown JJ, Wong BJ. (2009) Nondestructive imaging of live human keloid and facial tissue using multiphoton microscopy. Arch. Facial. Plast. Surg. 10(1):38-43.

[37] English RS, Shenefelt PD. (1999) Keloids and hypertrophic scars. *Dermatol. Surg*. 25(8):631-638. Review.

[38] Cicchi R, Kapsokalyvas D, De Giorgi V, Maio V, Van Wiechen A, Massi D, Lotti T, Pavone FS. (2010) Scoring of collagen organization in healthy and diseased human dermis by multiphoton microscopy. *J. Biophotonics*. 3(1-2):34-43.

[39] Bharati MH, Liu JJ, MacGregor J F. (2004) Image texture analysis: methods and comparisons. *Chemom. Intell. Lab. Syst*. 72(1):57-71.

[40] Castellano G, Bonilha L, Li LM, Cendes F. (2004) Texture analysis of medical images. *Clin. Radiol*. 59(12):1061-1069. Review.

[41] Wilhjelm JE, Grønholdt ML, Wiebe B, Jespersen SK, Hansen LK, Sillesen H. (1998) Quantitative analysis of ultrasound B-mode images of carotid atherosclerotic plaque: correlation with visual classification and histological examination. *IEEE Trans. Med. Imaging*. 17(6):910-922.

[42] Mahmoud-Ghoneim D, Toussaint G, Constans JM, de Certaines JD. (2003) Three dimensional texture analysis in MRI: a preliminary evaluation in gliomas. *Magn. Reson. Imaging*. 21(9):983-987.

[43] English RS, Shenefelt PD. (1999) Keloids and hypertrophic scars. *Dermatol. Surg*. 25:631–638.

[44] Walker RF, Jackway PT, Longstaff ID. (2003) Genetic Algorithm Optimisation of Adaptive Multi-Scale in GLCM Features. *Int. J. Pattern Recogn.* 17(1): 17–39.

[45] Hu W, Li H, Wang C, Gou S, Fu L. (2012) Characterization of collagen fibers by means of texture analysis of second harmonic generation images usingorientation-dependent gray level co-occurrence matrix method. *J. Biomed. Opt*. 17(2):026007.

Index

#

3D tissue scaffolds, viii, 2

A

accessibility, 74, 112
acetic acid, 6, 7, 11, 76
acetone, 34
acid, 6, 7, 14, 15, 19, 20, 31, 42, 43, 44, 53, 58, 75
acidic, 7, 9, 11, 20, 37
AD, 93, 113
adhesion, 27, 29, 55, 56, 60, 74
adipose, 35, 44
adipose tissue, 35
adsorption, 28, 37
adults, 112, 113
adverse conditions, 27
AFM, 18, 74
age, 15, 114
alanine, 15
allele, 93
alters, 33
amino, 4, 6, 13, 15, 17, 30, 45, 75, 93
amino acid(s), 4, 7, 13, 15, 17, 45, 93
amino groups, 30
ammonium, 12, 14, 33
antibiotic, 53
antibody, 49
Argentina, 87
arthroscope, 41, 43
articular cartilage, 41, 66
aseptic, 25
aspiration, 37
assessment, 13, 31, 41
atherosclerotic plaque, 115
atomic force, 46, 74
attachment, 26, 27, 34, 54
autosomal dominant, 93
autosomal recessive, 113

B

bacteria, 22, 74
basement membrane, 5
beams, 96
behaviors, viii, 27, 73
benefits, 95
bioactivity, vii, 1, 3, 16, 27, 28, 31, 49, 56
biocompatibility, vii, 1, 3, 6, 13, 21, 23, 26, 30, 31, 37, 42, 48, 56, 57, 63, 67, 70
biodegradability, 27
biodegradation, 22
biological properties, vii, 1, 48
biomarkers, 115
biomaterials, vii, viii, 1, 2, 3, 6, 12, 19, 21, 23, 25, 26, 28, 29, 32, 36, 41, 45, 48, 50
biomedical applications, 12, 50

biomolecules, 16
biopsy, ix, 88, 89, 98, 105, 111, 112, 114
biosafety, 2
biosynthesis, 4, 45, 50, 51, 92
blends, 30, 32
blood, 5, 23, 38, 40
blood transfusion, 23
blood vessels, 38, 40
body fluid, 23, 26
bonds, 58
bone(s), viii, 2, 25, 26, 27, 29, 30, 33, 34, 35, 36, 44, 47, 48, 52, 53, 54, 55, 57, 60, 70, 74, 88, 89, 93, 97, 110, 112
bone form, 29, 33
bone marrow, 36
bottom-up, 49
brain, 23
Brazil, 87, 104
breast cancer, 114
building blocks, 49

C

Ca^{2+}, 12
calcium, 29, 34, 59
capillary, 19, 75, 76, 78
capillary viscometry, 19
carbon, 29, 48, 55
carbon dioxide, 48
carboxyl, 6, 27, 30, 56
carcinogenicity, 22, 52
cartilage, viii, 2, 4, 25, 28, 30, 33, 36, 40, 41, 42, 43, 48, 57, 58, 64, 65, 66, 67, 70
cartilaginous, 40, 43
casting, 36, 61
cation, 12
cattle, 23
CBD, 30
cDNA, 48
cell biology, 44
cell culture, viii, 16, 30, 50, 61, 63, 73, 75, 83
cell differentiation, 44
cell line(s), 26, 48
cell scaffolds, viii, 73
cell surface, 76, 81
cellulose, 30, 57
ceramic, 27, 36, 61
challenges, 50
chemical(s), 4, 5, 6, 13, 16, 24, 28, 48
chemical reactions, 24
chicken, 75
China, 1
chitosan, 31, 34, 38, 39, 43, 48, 58, 59, 62, 70
Chitosan, 58, 63, 66
chondrocyte, 40, 42, 44, 48, 64, 65
chondroitin sulfate, 31
chromatography, 12
circular dichroism spectroscopy, vii, viii, 73
classification, viii, 2, 4, 12, 89, 101, 111, 115
cleavage, 92, 93
clinical application, 25, 26, 36, 40, 41, 50, 95, 97
clinical diagnosis, 110
clinical presentation, 112
clinical trials, 50
closure, 37
CMC, 38
coatings, viii, 2, 25, 53, 55
coding, viii, 88
coherence, 95
collaboration, 4
collage, 35
collagen sponges, 33, 58
collagen-based hydrogels, viii, 2, 4, 36, 39, 43
colon, 97, 98
colorectal cancer, 115
community, 105
compensation, 99
complement, 110
complexity, 16
complications, 33, 59
composites, 30, 33, 35, 58, 60
composition, 3, 12, 13, 18, 32, 34, 42, 57, 75
compression, 34, 37, 44, 61, 67
computational modeling, 71

condensation, 43
conditioning, 44
configuration, 99, 100
conjugation, 49
connective tissue, vii, viii, ix, 1, 2, 25, 40, 53, 69, 74, 88, 92, 93, 97
consensus, 13
conserving, 95
constituents, 40
construction, 4, 30
contamination, 99
copolymer, 53
copper, 6
cornea, 31, 39, 58, 97
correlation, 41, 55, 97, 104, 105, 108, 110, 111, 115
cortical bone, 33, 58, 114
cost, 5, 12
cryopreservation, 28
crystalline, 37
crystallization, 37
culture, 26, 29, 34, 36, 41, 42, 43, 44, 48, 67, 77, 81, 82
culture conditions, 44
culture medium, 81
cysteine, 114
cytocompatibility, 26, 34, 37
cytotoxicity, 21, 51

D

database, 75, 113
decay, 93, 108, 110, 111, 113
defects, 33, 35, 36, 41, 43, 45, 57, 58, 65, 93, 105
deficiencies, 26
deficiency, 88
deformation, 19, 89, 110
degradation, 22, 31, 34, 52, 57
denaturation, 17, 76, 82
deposition, 26, 28, 95
depth, 95, 111
derivatives, 45
dermis, 29, 38, 47, 97, 98, 100, 105, 107, 108, 110, 112, 115
detection, 14, 19, 23, 24, 91, 115
diabetes, 33, 59
dialysis, 11, 12, 37, 61
diarrhea, 24
differential scanning, vii, viii, 73, 75, 76, 83
differential scanning calorimeter, 76
differential scanning calorimetry, vii, viii, 73, 75, 83
diffraction, 46
digestion, 6, 7, 8, 9, 24
discrimination, 101
disease model, 47
diseases, 23, 97, 112
disorder, 92, 97
dispersion, 19, 99
dissociation, 17
dissociation temperature, 17
distribution, 6, 19, 32, 34, 47, 69, 91
DOI, 69
dressings, 37
drug delivery, 3
drug release, 53
drugs, 35
drying, 33, 34
DSC, 17, 75, 76, 78, 79, 82, 83
dyeing, 14
dysplasia, 89

E

ECM, 38, 43, 58, 93
Ehlers-Danlos syndrome, 114
elastin, 15, 33, 39, 56, 58, 59, 63, 96
electric field, 95
electrochemical deposition, 28, 53
electrolyte, 6
electron, 76, 81
electrophoresis, 14
electrospinning, 26, 28, 30, 33, 35
embossing, 33, 58
embryonic stem cells, 26, 38, 44
emission, 95, 115
encephalopathy, 23
encoding, 48, 93
endothelial cells, 27, 39, 53

endotoxins, 15
energy, 27, 91, 95, 103, 104, 105, 106, 107, 110, 111
engineering, 26, 28, 29, 31, 34, 36, 37, 39, 40, 42, 48, 49, 50, 61, 67
environment(s), ix, 2, 5, 9, 24, 35, 36, 38, 44, 62, 88, 89, 94
enzyme(s), 4, 6, 7, 9, 14, 20, 40, 55, 93
enzyme immobilization, 55
epidemic, 23
epidermis, 5, 37, 100
epithelial cells, 39
epithelium, 39, 99
equilibrium, 78
ESCs, 26
ESD, 28
ester, 49
estrogen, 47
ethanol, 6, 24
ethylene, 6, 24, 38, 49
ethylene glycol, 38
ethylene oxide, 24, 49
evaporation, 37
evidence, 81, 83
evolution, 99
examinations, 89
excision, 105
excitation, 91, 95, 96, 99
exclusion, 12
exocytosis, 92
experimental condition, 43
exposure, 20, 22, 41
extracellular matrix, 17, 25, 26, 32, 36, 40, 42, 46, 50, 61, 69, 74, 88, 89, 92, 93, 95
extraction, vii, 2, 4, 5, 6, 7, 8, 9, 10, 11
extrusion, 33

F

fabrication, viii, 2, 26, 34, 35, 36, 38, 43, 45, 47, 54, 58, 59, 60, 61, 62
fat, 5, 60
female rat, 53
fetus, 89
fiber(s), vii, viii, ix, 4, 5, 16, 17, 18, 19, 26, 28, 33, 34, 35, 46, 47, 49, 55, 59, 69, 88, 91, 94, 97, 98, 100, 101, 102, 103, 104, 105, 106, 107, 108, 110, 111, 116
fiber bundles, 5, 97, 102
fibrils, vii, viii, ix, 17, 36, 39, 47, 61, 69, 73, 74, 75, 76, 81, 83, 88, 91, 92, 93, 94, 95, 97, 114
fibrin, 43, 62
fibroblast growth factor, 35, 43, 45, 60
fibroblast proliferation, 36
fibroblasts, ix, 28, 38, 39, 88, 89, 112
fibrosis, 97
fibrous cap, 43
fibrous tissue, vii, 1
films, 13, 24, 27, 28, 29, 30, 31, 32, 53, 56, 57
filters, 16
filtration, 24
fish, 48
fixation, 41, 111
fluctuations, 74, 102
fluid, 37
fluorescence, 95, 96, 99, 114, 115
fluorophores, 49
force, 36, 47
formation, viii, 28, 37, 46, 49, 55, 59, 61, 74, 77, 78, 79, 81, 82, 92
formula, 109
fractures, 88, 90, 110
fragility, viii, 88, 110
France, 48
freezing, 33, 34, 59
FTIR, 18
functionalization, 56

G

gamma radiation, 13
ganglion, 34
gel, 14, 16, 36, 43, 61, 63, 66
gene expression, 29, 42, 43
genes, viii, 19, 40, 88, 93, 105
genetic background, 24
genetic information, 97, 110

genotype, 93, 97
Germany, 99, 100
gingival, 29
glucose, 33
glue, 43
glycine, 15, 93
glycosaminoglycans, 15
granules, 9
growth, 15, 30, 32, 34, 35, 43, 44, 46, 67, 75, 88, 89
growth factor, 30, 32, 35, 43, 44, 67
growth rate, 75
guidelines, 12, 21, 24
Guinea, 22
hyaline, 40
hybrid, 37, 38, 63, 65
hybridization, 49
hydrogels, viii, 2, 4, 14, 24, 25, 36, 37, 38, 39, 42, 43, 44, 49, 62, 63, 67, 68
hydrogen, 15
hydrogen bonds, 15
hydrolysis, 27
hydrolyzed collagen, 15, 75, 83
hydroxide, 33
hydroxyapatite, 27, 34, 45, 48, 50, 55, 59, 68, 70
hypersensitivity, 23
hypoxia, 43, 66

H

hair, 5, 105
hair follicle, 5, 105
hazards, 48
HE, 113
healing, 26, 40, 45, 97
hearing loss, 89
heating rate, 76, 78
heavy metals, 6, 16
helicity, vii, viii, 73, 82, 83
hemostasis, 46, 69, 74
herpes, 24
herpes virus, 24
heterogeneity, 97, 112
HFP, 30
histochemistry, 44
histological examination, 115
histology, 49
history, 25, 26, 29, 41
homogeneity, 102, 104, 105, 111
host, 15, 29
hot spots, 103
human, vii, ix, 1, 2, 3, 16, 21, 23, 25, 26, 29, 32, 33, 34, 35, 36, 38, 40, 42, 44, 46, 48, 55, 59, 62, 63, 67, 68, 70, 88, 91, 97, 98, 100, 102, 110, 111, 112, 113, 114, 115
human body, vii, 1, 25, 40
human skin, ix, 88, 91, 98, 110, 111, 112, 113, 114

I

ID, 116
ideal, vii, 1, 4, 17, 31, 38, 40, 43, 49
identification, 22, 52, 110
image(s), 17, 91, 94, 97, 98, 99, 100, 101, 102, 103, 104, 105, 106, 107, 108, 110, 111, 114, 115, 116
immersion, 99
immobilization, 27, 54
immunocompromised, 29
immunogenicity, 21
immunohistochemistry, 44, 49
implants, 21, 26, 28, 62
improvements, viii, 2, 41, 112
impurities, 11, 15
in vitro, 16, 21, 26, 28, 30, 37, 38, 39, 40, 41, 43, 44, 45, 48, 49, 51, 54, 56, 59, 63, 67, 74, 75
in vivo, 4, 6, 16, 23, 26, 30, 35, 37, 39, 44, 55, 67, 98, 101
incidence, 92
incubation period, 77, 83
incubation time, 76, 77, 81
induction, 55
industry, 19
inflammation, 29
ingestion, 23
injury, 39, 46
insertion, 93

insulin, 43
integration, 35, 43, 46
integrins, 112
integrity, 43, 50, 74
interface, 28, 100
interference, 14
intermolecular interactions, 74
intrinsic viscosity, 19
ions, 12
irradiation, 24
Islam, 62
isolation, 98
Israel, 48
issues, 23

J

Japan, 73, 75, 76

K

K^+, 12
keratinocyte(s), 29, 30
keratoplasty, 39
kinetic parameters, 81
kinetics, 9, 55, 75, 77

L

lactic acid, 30, 53, 57
lasers, 99
leaching, 56
lead, 6, 13, 24, 89
lens, 99
lesions, 41
ligament(s), vii, viii, 1, 2, 74
light, ix, 88, 94, 95, 99, 100
lipids, 15

M

magnesium, 27
magnetic field, 39
magnetic resonance, 41, 42, 89
magnetic resonance imaging, 41, 42, 89
majority, 97
mammal, 25
mammalian cells, 22
manufacturing, 24
mapping, 42, 68
marine fish, 48
marrow, 68
mass, 9
materials, vii, viii, ix, 1, 2, 3, 5, 15, 21, 23, 26, 27, 29, 32, 35, 41, 44, 61, 88, 94, 95
matrix, 5, 6, 27, 32, 38, 41, 42, 43, 44, 47, 50, 54, 56, 59, 65, 91, 97, 101, 102, 103, 107, 108, 109, 116
matter, 13, 14
measurement(s), 14, 17, 19, 69, 75, 76, 77, 78, 79, 80, 82, 89, 102, 112
mechanical properties, 24, 27, 30, 35, 37, 39, 43, 44, 66, 67
mechanical stress, 33, 59
mediation, 42
medical, vii, viii, 2, 12, 21, 22, 23, 24, 26, 42, 47, 50, 51, 52, 101, 105, 115
medicine, 52
melting, 76, 79, 80, 82
melting temperature, 76
membranes, viii, 2, 13, 24, 25, 28, 29, 31, 32, 57, 58
mercury, 6
mesenchymal stem cells, 27, 36, 48, 50, 53, 55, 67, 68
metals, 6, 26
meter, 34
Mg^{2+}, 12
mice, 29, 55
microenvironments, 74
microgravity, 39
microscope, 76, 89, 99, 100
microscopy, vii, ix, 46, 69, 74, 88, 89, 91, 94, 95, 98, 99, 100, 103, 110, 111, 112, 113, 114, 115
microspheres, 25, 27, 35, 53, 60
microstructure(s), 46, 61, 69
migration, 12, 19, 29, 53

mineralization, 44, 55
mixing, 6, 8
MMP(s), 42, 49
models, 47, 49, 53, 74
modifications, 32, 40, 94
modules, 29, 55
modulus, 33, 34, 36, 38
moisture, 13
moisture content, 13
molds, 33
molecular biology, 62
molecular structure, 69
molecular weight, 6, 11, 19, 75, 76
molecular weight distribution, 6, 11, 19
molecules, vii, viii, 15, 16, 28, 30, 49, 50, 73, 74, 77, 81, 82, 92, 93, 95, 96
monolayer, 26
monomers, 37, 46
morphology, 19, 28, 35, 47, 76, 81, 82, 91, 101, 104
MRI, 41, 64, 89, 116
mRNA, 40, 93
multiwalled carbon nanotubes, 29
muscles, 5
musculoskeletal, 66
mutation(s), viii, 22, 88, 90, 92, 93, 94, 105, 112, 113
myocardium, 30, 62

N

Na^+, 12
NaCl, 8
nanocomposites, 34, 37, 52
nanofibers, 33, 35, 49, 59
nanofibrous membranes, 30
nanoparticles, 40, 49, 63, 71
nanotube, 55
National Academy of Sciences, 66, 68
natural polymers, 25, 42, 45
nerve, 35, 40, 60, 63
nerve growth factor, 40, 63
nervous system, 23
neurons, 34
neutral, viii, 6, 7, 11, 12, 14, 73, 79, 83
neutrophils, 74, 77, 81
NH2, 27
NHS, 31, 39
nonlinear optics, 115

O

obstacles, 25
OECD, 22
OI disorders, ix, 88
oil, 99
optimism, 97
organ(s), 4, 5, 16, 35, 93, 94, 97
organism, 93
osteocyte, 45
Osteogenesis, v, viii, 87, 88, 90, 92, 112, 113
osteogenesis imperfecta, viii, 88, 93, 112, 113, 114
osteoporosis, 89, 92, 93
ovarian cancer, 115
ovarian tumor, 115
overlap, 17, 46, 47

P

parallel, 92, 97
parathyroid, 45, 68
parathyroid hormone, 45, 68
pass/fail, 12
pathogens, 74
pathologist, 111
PCR, 44
pepsin, 6, 7, 9, 24, 75, 83
peptide(s), 6, 7, 30, 38, 49, 71, 74, 93
pericardium, 32
perinatal, 90, 93
periodicity, 17, 111
periodontal, 29
periosteum, 41
permeability, 35, 37
pH, viii, 7, 9, 11, 20, 24, 73, 75, 76, 77, 78, 79, 80, 81, 82, 83
phenol, 14

phenotype(s), 25, 31, 42, 93, 97, 110, 114
phosphate, 34, 44, 59, 61, 67, 75, 76, 77, 78, 80
phosphates, 45
photons, 91, 95
physical and mechanical properties, 33
physical properties, 28, 34, 54, 56
plants, 48, 70, 71
polarity, 91, 113
polarization, 95
poly(N-vinylpyrrolidone), 28
polyacrylamide, 14
polymer(s), 12, 19, 26, 27, 35, 39, 42, 43, 49, 52, 55, 66, 71
polymeric materials, 42
polymerization, 43
polypeptide(s), 13, 19, 20, 24, 33, 49, 58
polystyrene, 28
polyurethane, 28, 55
polyvinyl alcohol, 37
population, 40, 96
porosity, 54, 59
precipitation, 8, 11, 12
pregnancy, 112
preparation, vii, 2, 3, 4, 12, 13, 16, 18, 19, 20, 23, 24, 28, 30, 33, 36, 41, 45, 46, 48, 50, 54, 58, 77, 80
preservation, 33
principles, 104
probability, 101, 102
probability density function, 102
probe, 17, 95
progenitor cells, 38, 62
proliferation, 27, 28, 29, 31, 35, 39, 43, 53, 54, 74
proline, 15
proteins, 11, 12, 17, 26, 35, 39, 42, 63, 92
proteoglycans, 40, 112
prototype, 56
pulp, 40, 63
purification, vii, 2, 4, 8, 11, 24
purity, 14, 19
PVA, 37

Q

quality control, 19
quantification, ix, 22, 52, 88, 97, 98, 103, 106, 112

R

raw materials, 3, 4, 9, 23, 24
RE, 113
reaction rate, 9
reactions, 6
reactivity, 22, 57
reagents, 14
recession, 29
reconstruction, viii, 2, 4, 27, 30, 62, 111
recovery, 39, 41
regeneration, vii, viii, 2, 25, 26, 29, 30, 33, 34, 35, 37, 38, 40, 42, 43, 44, 46, 48, 50, 52, 54, 56, 57, 58, 60, 62, 65, 68
regenerative medicine, vii, viii, 73
regulations, 23
rehabilitation, 26, 41
repair, 29, 39, 40, 41, 42, 45, 48, 57, 68
reparation, viii, 2
requirements, 12, 13, 22, 23, 33, 35
researchers, 27, 40, 48, 75
residues, 7, 17
resilience, 50
resolution, 11, 19, 75, 76, 89, 91, 99, 111, 113
response, 6, 28, 29, 31, 35, 36, 42, 54, 55, 68, 74, 95, 98
reticulum, 92, 93
risk(s), viii, 2, 4, 21, 23, 48, 50, 51
risk management, 21, 51
RNA, 113
rodents, 22
room temperature, 28, 77
root(s), 5, 34, 103
roughness, 31
rutile, 27

S

safety, 23
salts, 7, 11, 12
scanning electron microscopy, 74, 83
scar tissue, vii, 1
scatter, 96
scattering, 96, 98
science, 45, 71
SDS-PAGE, 14, 19
Second Harmonic Generation, ix, 88
seeding, viii, 39, 43, 74, 81, 83
self-assembly, 16, 43, 49, 51, 71, 74, 75, 77, 78, 79, 81, 82
SEM micrographs, 81, 82
sensitivity, 91, 97
sensitization, 22, 51
septum, 48
serum, 14, 83
serum albumin, 14
shape, 19, 24
shelf life, 13, 20
SHG, vii, ix, 46, 69, 88, 91, 94, 95, 96, 97, 98, 99, 100, 101, 102, 103, 104, 105, 106, 107, 108, 110, 111, 112
showing, viii, 27, 34, 49, 74, 94, 96, 106
side chain, 17, 74
signal peptide, 7
signals, ix, 88, 94, 99, 108, 114
signs, 89
silica, 37, 52
silk, 34, 42, 45, 60, 68
silver, 6
simulation(s), 9, 10, 27, 35, 53, 97, 113
sintering, 42
skin, vii, viii, 1, 2, 4, 5, 6, 7, 8, 9, 15, 22, 25, 26, 29, 37, 48, 49, 51, 52, 54, 59, 74, 75, 88, 91, 93, 94, 97, 99, 100, 101, 104, 105, 106, 107, 108, 110, 111, 112, 115
small intestine, 30
small-angle scattering, 113
SO42-, 12
sodium, 6, 7, 12, 14, 39, 75, 76, 78
software, 47, 76, 79, 99
sol-gel, 37
solubility, 11, 50
solution, 6, 7, 9, 11, 12, 14, 15, 19, 20, 21, 24, 26, 34, 37, 46, 75, 76, 78, 105
solvents, 33
SP, 100, 104, 114
species, 21, 49
spectrophotometric method, 16
spectrophotometry, 14
spectroscopy, vii, viii, 73
sponge, 13, 27, 32, 33, 34, 35, 36, 44, 48, 53, 70
stability, 15, 17, 19, 37, 39, 51, 69, 75, 78
stabilization, viii, 49, 73
starch, 35
state(s), viii, 2, 76, 78, 95, 96, 97, 113
stem cell differentiation, 55
stem cells, 26, 40, 44, 63
stimulation, 44
storage, 20, 36
stroma, 39, 89
stromal cells, 39, 59
structural changes, 97
structural protein, vii, 1, 2, 25, 92, 93, 113
structural variation, 111
structure, viii, ix, 3, 4, 6, 7, 13, 15, 16, 17, 18, 19, 21, 24, 29, 32, 33, 34, 36, 40, 44, 45, 47, 50, 51, 53, 55, 58, 59, 68, 69, 73, 74, 75, 79, 81, 82, 88, 92, 94, 97, 103, 104, 108
subacute, 22, 23
subcutaneous tissue, 29
submucosa, 30
substitutes, 37, 59
substitution(s), 93, 114
substrate(s), 9, 21, 23, 26, 27, 28, 35, 42, 45, 53, 55
sulfate, 12, 14, 34, 42, 43, 44, 66
sulfur, 15
Sun, 114, 115
supervision, 23
surface coatings, viii, 2, 25
surface modification, 3, 26, 28
surface properties, 57
surfactants, 6
surgical technique, 41

survival, 29, 34, 55
susceptibility, 88, 95, 115
Sweden, 40
Switzerland, 51, 52
symbiosis, 5
symmetry, 46, 95
syndrome, 113
synthesis, 49, 59
synthetic polymers, 27, 42

T

tantalum, 27, 53
target, 6
technical assistance, 83
techniques, 2, 17, 33, 41, 50, 89, 91, 96, 97, 110, 111
technology, 28, 39, 99
teeth, 47
TEM, 17, 51
temperature, 11, 17, 33, 46, 68, 75, 76, 78, 79
tendon(s), vii, 1, 4, 47, 51, 60, 74, 88, 91, 97, 113, 114
tensile strength, 30, 31, 33, 34, 42
testing, 21, 51
texture, 91, 101, 102, 103, 104, 105, 107, 110, 111, 112, 115, 116
thermal stability, 4, 15, 16, 37, 74, 79, 81, 82, 83
thermodynamic equilibrium, 76
thermodynamic parameters, 76
thermograms, 78, 79
thermogravimetric analysis, 14
thin films, 25, 55, 57
tin, 6
tissue engineering, viii, 2, 3, 23, 24, 25, 27, 29, 31, 32, 33, 34, 35, 36, 37, 38, 39, 40, 41, 45, 47, 48, 49, 50, 52, 53, 54, 55, 56, 57, 58, 59, 60, 61, 63, 65, 66, 68, 70
titanium, 26, 28, 53
TNF, 42
tobacco, 48, 70
topology, 46
toxicity, 22, 51, 52
toxicology, 23
trachea, 39
transformations, 112
transforming growth factor, 34, 59
transition temperature, 17, 75, 76
translation, 92
Transmission Electron Microscopy (TEM), 17
transparency, 39
transplantation, 42
transport, 92
trauma, 88
treatment, 6, 12, 24, 40, 41, 43, 65, 110
tryptophan, 15
turnover, 47
type I collagen, vii, viii, 1, 2, 3, 4, 7, 13, 14, 15, 19, 21, 23, 24, 25, 27, 32, 37, 38, 46, 47, 50, 66, 67, 68, 69, 70, 75, 88, 92, 112, 113, 114
Type I collagen, vii, viii, 1, 26, 62, 68, 73, 74, 88, 93

U

ultrasonography, 89
ultrasound, 46, 69, 89, 115
ultrastructure, viii, 69, 73, 95
umbilical cord, 44, 67
uniform, 34
United States, 16, 66, 68
USA, 68, 99
UV, 17

V

valve, 32
variations, 104
vascular endothelial growth factor (VEGF), 30
vascularization, 30
vein, 29
velocity, 99
vertebrates, 50
vessels, 5

viral pathogens, 24
viruses, 16, 48
viscoelastic properties, 49
viscosity, 7, 9, 19, 20, 24
visualization, 82

W

water, 6, 11, 13, 14, 28, 36, 37
water vapor, 37
WD, 99
weakness, 27
Western blot, 16
worldwide, 40
wound healing, vii, 1, 56, 97

X

X-ray diffraction, 46
X-ray diffraction data, 46

Y

yield, 5, 6